The Yoga Doctor

Patti Shelton, MD

ISBN 978-0-9965329-0-7

NOTICE

This book is intended to be used for informational purposes only. It is not intended to diagnose, prevent, or treat any medical condition. It is not a substitute for qualified professional medical advice. For diagnosis or treatment of any medical condition, consult your own doctor.

This book does not create a doctor/patient relationship between the author and the reader, and no such relationship is implied.

The author assumes no responsibility for any health condition that requires medical supervision, and is not liable for any damages or negative consequences created by following the information in this book. Consult with your doctor before beginning a yoga practice, or before making changes in your yoga practice, to ensure that you are taking the most appropriate actions for your specific situation.

While the author has made all reasonable efforts to ensure the accuracy of the information presented herein, the author and the publisher do not assume and hereby completely disclaim any liability to any party caused by errors or omissions.

CONTENTS

Introduction..1
Section 1: Body Structures..5
Chapter 1: Connective Tissue..7
Chapter 2: Joints...17
Chapter 3: Muscles...25
Chapter 4: Safe vs. Unsafe Sensations..................................37
Section 2: The Spine..45
Chapter 5: Posture..47
Chapter 6: The Neck...67
Chapter 7: The Low Back..83
Section 3: The Arms...101
Chapter 8: The Shoulders..103
Chapter 9: The Elbows..123
Chapter 10: The Wrists and Hands......................................135
Section 4: The Legs...145
Chapter 11: The Hips...147
Chapter 12: The Knees..171
Chapter 13: The Ankles and Feet..191
Conclusion: Yoga Inspiration..207

INTRODUCTION

Have you ever heard one of these comments?

"Downward dog hurts my wrists."

"I meditate in lotus pose, but my knees ache afterward."

"My shoulders get sore in child's pose."

The most common response from yoga teachers? "Keep working on your flexibility. One day, you'll be open enough to get the pose."

Maybe. Either that, or the student will get osteoarthritis.

And these are the students who are lucky enough to experience pain while they're damaging their joints. Others may not know how much they're hurting themselves until years later. They may not ever find out what caused their problems. As a medical doctor and a yoga teacher, I find this situation tragic.

Yoga can be an incredible tool to stay healthy and live a long life. New research studies continue to be added to the pile of proof that yoga is good for you. Avoiding yoga because you're worried about injury is not the answer. The answer is to empower yourself with knowledge.

It's unfortunate that most yoga teachers – let alone yoga students –

aren't trained very thoroughly in anatomy. Students tend to assume that their teachers have expertise in this area, but unfortunately, that's often not the case. Most yoga teacher trainings focus on handing down the "classic" forms of the poses.

The ancient masters of yoga had incredible knowledge of many valuable things. One thing they didn't know much about was biomechanics. Lacking a thorough knowledge of how the body is put together inside, and generally aiming to transcend the body in any case, they developed the practice with very little attention to the possible long-term harm.

We can learn from these masters while still getting the benefit of modern scientific insight into how the body works and how to protect it.

If you're a yoga teacher, you probably feel the burden of responsibility for keeping your students safe. You became a yoga teacher to promote health and wellness. The last thing you want is to cause injuries. But do you know how to avoid them?

If you're a yoga student (and all yoga teachers are students too), you probably came to yoga for your health and longevity. Maybe you wanted a stronger, leaner, more agile body; maybe you were attracted to the holistic mind-body focus of yoga. You probably heard that yoga was a safe form of exercise, which it is, when practiced appropriately.

The key is to learn how to protect yourself – and, if you're a teacher, your students. The "classic" forms of many poses may work for some bodies, but can cause injury to others.

Some people avoid yoga because of the pain they experience. Others continue with the practice because of its many benefits, pushing through the pain and causing chronic joint damage. Either outcome is incredibly unfortunate, when minor modifications could have helped them to protect themselves. Just a little knowledge can make all the difference.

The careers of ballet dancers and gymnasts often end by their 30s due to damage to their joints. Unfortunately, multiple surgeries and chronic pain are not uncommon in this population. By contrast, many famous yogis continued to practice into their 80s and 90s. Don't you want to be one of them?

As a medical doctor, I know the body inside and out. And as a yoga teacher, I know the practice. I frequently lead workshops and trainings on these topics. I'm passionate about helping people practice yoga safely.

This book was born from the "aha!" moments of my students. When they figure out why a pose hurts every time they do it, and find out how damaging it could be to continue doing it the painful way, they can't believe they'd never learned this information before.

I've made everything as simple as possible, without "dumbing it down" at all. I know that long, dry anatomy texts make most people's eyes cross. If you're allergic to long Latin and Greek words, don't worry – this book is hypoallergenic. Tamsin, a student in a yoga teacher training course I taught, told me that she'd taken multiple anatomy courses before, but mine was the first one she actually understood.

When I take other teachers' yoga classes, I notice how frequently the cues are unsafe for many people's bodies. Everyone is entitled to their own way of doing things, of course; and as you'll see, I don't insist on a "one-size-fits-all" approach. But I'm also sure that yoga teachers don't want to be hurting their students, and I'm even more sure that yoga students don't want to deal with injuries.

What are you doing in your yoga practice that's damaging your joints? Do you even know that you're hurting yourself? The short time it will take you to read this book will pay off in every single yoga class you take – or teach – for the rest of your life.

The huge benefits of yoga can be yours, without the risk of long-term injury. This book will teach you how.

SECTION 1:
BODY STRUCTURES

What is a ligament, and can I stretch it safely? Why do my muscles quiver in certain poses, and should I be concerned when they do that? How can I figure out which sensations are safe and which ones indicate that I'm damaging my body?

This section will answer these and many more questions. We'll explore the structures that make up the human body, including connective tissue, joints, and muscles. Then I'll present the basic framework for knowing what various bodily sensations mean and which ones are safe.

Let's dive in.

CHAPTER 1:
CONNECTIVE TISSUE

There is a web of tissue throughout the body that physically binds it together. Through this structure, the body is connected and made continuous, a true whole rather than a set of parts. In keeping with its function, this tissue is called connective tissue.

If you want to understand why certain types of movement are safe and others are unsafe, then it's essential to have a basic understanding of how your connective tissue is structured. Connective tissue can be put at risk by certain ways of moving the body. That's why we're beginning this book by exploring the structure of this type of tissue.

Connective tissue is one of four basic types of tissues in the body:

- Muscle tissue
- Nervous tissue
- Epithelial tissue
- Connective tissue

Muscle tissue is pretty self-explanatory. Nervous tissue refers to the nervous system (think "nerves"). Epithelial tissue is the skin and the linings of things (such as the respiratory tract and digestive tract).

Everything else is connective tissue. There's a lot of "everything else" in your body, including some things you might not initially think of as connective tissue. All of these are connective tissue:

- Ligaments
- Tendons
- Cartilage
- Fascia
- Bone
- Adipose tissue (fat)

These seemingly disparate things aren't grouped together simply because of the tendency of scientists to want to group things. (Although, undoubtedly, scientists do have an abiding love for creating categories.) These types of tissue share a basic common structure at the smallest level. Let's zoom in to see what makes them similar.

What is Connective Tissue Made Of?

Most tissues are made up primarily of cells, the "building blocks of life." Connective tissue is different. It does contain cells, but relatively few of them. It's mainly made up of two other things, both of which are outside the cells: fibers and ground substance.

Fibers, as their name suggests, are generally long, thin molecules that give connective tissue most of its structure and strength. The type of fibers differs from one connective tissue to the next. The most common is Type I collagen, which constitutes about 25% of all of the protein in your body. There are other types of collagen, and also other similar proteins that can serve this function.

Ground substances are small molecules that act to hold water in a tissue, keeping it moist. The most common one in most types of connective tissue is hyaluronic acid, although some connective tissues have other types (for instance, in bone, the ground substance is mineralized). The ground substance is similar to a gel, ensuring that the connective tissue is hydrated and yet can hold its shape.

Those are the things that connective tissue does contain. Also very important are the things it doesn't contain, at least not in large amounts. Most connective tissues contain very few blood vessels (bones being a notable exception to this). With few cells to do repair work, and little blood flow to bring in new cells and nutrients, connective tissue has a difficult time healing if it's injured. Often, injured connective tissue never heals fully.

Also, while certain types of connective tissue contain many nerve endings, others have very few. Nerve endings are the parts of nerves that are sensitive; with only a few of them, there isn't always pain when connective tissue is being damaged. Cartilage is a notable example of this lack of innervation. Particularly with the kind of insidious damage that can occur slowly over a long period of time, there may be little sensation of pain until years into the process.

This is why it's so important to practice yoga (and do other activities) safely. We don't want to injure tissues that can't fully heal. We might not always feel pain when we're hurting ourselves. Worst of all, the consequences of damaging our connective tissues can significantly affect our quality of life.

Now, let's look at some specific types of connective tissue, to find out more specifics about each one and how to protect it.

Ligaments

Ligaments connect a bone to another bone, acting to stabilize a joint. They're important in the protection of a joint, because they prevent it from moving in ways that could damage it. When the ligaments are unable to adequately perform their function, the joint may deteriorate, potentially leading to osteoarthritis.

Ligaments are primarily made up of Type I collagen. The collagen molecule is a triple helix, made up of three strands of protein wound around each other, like a rope. Imagine many of these ropes end to end, creating a long fiber. Now, imagine many of these long fibers placed next to each other. That's the structure of ligaments.

In order to hold all of those strands in place, the collagen molecules form molecular bonds known as "cross-links" with the collagen molecules next to them. It's like adjacent ropes being tied together with strings. This keeps the collagen molecules from sliding past each other, giving the ligament its strength.

Now imagine trying to stretch this structure. The collagen fibers are already nearly straight, so they can't be stretched very much. That means the only way to stretch the ligament or tendon is to pull the collagen molecules past each other. This breaks the cross-linkages between them.

Unfortunately, once broken, these cross-linkages don't form again very efficiently; if they do form, they may do so in the new, longer shape of the ligament. In other words, once stretched, ligaments will generally stay stretched. Because ligaments protect a joint by preventing it from moving in damaging ways, stretching them leaves the joint more vulnerable to damage. (Interestingly, the formation of too many cross-linkages between collagen molecules is thought to contribute to disease processes like the stiffening of arterial walls.)

Ligaments lack a good blood supply, and heal very slowly. They may never heal completely after an injury. However, ligaments do contain nerve endings, which detect stretch and will signal excessive stretch with pain. This allows you to know when you're stretching your ligaments too far, so you can protect your joints. When we discuss specific joints, we'll explore which sensations indicate that you're stretching the ligaments, so you know when to back off.

Tendons

Tendons and ligaments are very similar to each other on a microscopic level, but they exist in different locations. While ligaments connect a bone to a bone, tendons connect a muscle to a bone, allowing muscle contractions to pull on the bones and cause movement.

Tendons have a few differences from ligaments. Due to a slight difference in their collagen makeup, they have some ability to stretch, although it's quite limited in most tendons (at most 15% of their length, and often more like half of that). This allows some tendons to store part of the energy produced by a muscle contraction, and then release it to cause movement. However, the stretching ability is still limited, and overstretching tendons can cause them to become permanently lengthened.

Like ligaments, tendons have almost no blood supply, so the healing process of an injured tendon is slow and may be incomplete; however, they do contain nerve endings. Fortunately, this allows you to detect potential danger to your tendons and act to protect them.

Fascia

The fascia (FASH-uh) wrap around a muscle in many layers. We'll look more at these layers in Chapter 3; for now, let's consider the microscopic structure of fascia.

Fascia contains collagen, too, but it also contains a protein that's different in important ways. This protein is called elastin, and its name gives a clue as to its nature; it's elastic. Picture the elastin molecule as a wavy line instead of a straight one. These wavy lines are inserted among all of those straight collagen lines.

When stretching, the wavy line has an advantage. It can stretch out to become straight without breaking any of its cross-linkages with other neighboring molecules. When the stretch is released, the elastin simply bounces back into its original shape. (On a molecular level, this is pretty much how elastic works.) That means fascia can be stretched much farther than can tendons or ligaments, without becoming permanently lax.

Bone

The image of bones in the popular media is similar to that of rocks; they're just big chunks of mineral that get pushed around by other things. When we see a dry old bone, it looks white and very rock-like, reinforcing this idea.

While dead bones may be similar to rocks, living bones are completely different. A living bone doesn't even look white at all; it looks pink, because of all of the blood flowing through it. Unusually among connective tissues, bone is extremely vascularized (meaning that it has lots of blood vessels) and also extremely innervated (meaning that it has lots of nerves).

The inner part of a bone is hollow; during childhood, the bone is filled with red bone marrow, which makes blood cells. (During adulthood, most of the red marrow has been replaced by "yellow marrow," which is actually not bone marrow at all, but fat.) Surrounding the outside of the bone is a covering of connective tissue called the periosteum, which is structurally similar to tendon.

When a bone breaks, it hurts – a lot. That's because of all the nerves in the bone. However, because bone is so vascular, this type of injury will heal quite well in healthy people. (Though the bone will not, as the urban myth claims, be stronger than it was before it broke.)

Bones are also continually remodeled in response to the forces placed upon them. Within the bone tissue are several types of bone cells. One type of cell is always breaking down bone tissue, while another is always building it up; the balance between these two determines how strong the bone will be.

When force is placed on a bone (i.e., during weight-bearing exercise), the cells that build bone tissue are stimulated, and the bone gets stronger. The fibers and minerals in the bone are laid down in a pattern that allows the bone optimally to handle the forces it regularly experiences. If you want to have strong bones, do weight-bearing exercise! Otherwise, the cells that break down bone tissue will slowly win, making fractures more likely as you age. You can lift weights, or do body weight exercises like yoga, but this really is a use-it-or-lose-it situation. (Any exercise where you're using your strength to hold up your body weight will work; in yoga, warrior poses, chair pose, and plank are examples.)

When you're a child, your bones contain cartilage plates from which the bones grow. During this time, the shape of your bones is malleable. However, at puberty, the cartilage plates become bone tissue (they "fuse" or "ossify"), and the shape of the bones becomes more or less set. After that, while the bone gets stronger or weaker based on how it's used, its shape isn't going to change very much.

As we'll see, the shape of your bones determines how much safe range of motion you'll have at each joint. Because bone shapes are essentially set at puberty, it's important to honor the limitations imposed by your bones. Attempts to change your bones' shapes will not succeed, and can cause damage.

Cartilage

While the strong mineralized tissue of bone is ideal in many parts of the body, there are other places where flexibility is necessary along with strength. This is where cartilage comes in. It's a strong material, but is also malleable.

There are three types of cartilage: elastic cartilage, hyaline cartilage, and fibrocartilage. These vary in the proportion of elastin to collagen that they contain, with elastic cartilage being the most flexible and fibrocartilage being the stiffest. As we'll soon explore, hyaline cartilage plays a significant role in the synovial joints of the body, and its health is crucial to keeping your joints pain-free.

Cartilage is completely avascular, meaning that it has no blood supply. The cells within the tissue get their nutrients and rid their waste products via diffusion into the surrounding fluids. This makes cartilage extremely vulnerable to damage, because effective healing is almost impossible without a blood supply. Because it also lacks significant innervation, damage to the cartilage can sometimes go undetected. We'll be talking throughout this book about keeping the cartilage of all of your joints healthy.

Hypermobility

There are genetic components to flexibility, related to small differences in the structures of proteins such as collagen. Certain people are dramatically more flexible than average, because their connective tissue is structured differently. This is known as hyperflexibility, or hypermobility.

It can be dangerous for an average person to watch a hypermobile person practice yoga. When you see someone who's extremely flexible go through a yoga sequence, it's common to think, "One day I'll be able to do that. I'm going to work really hard in yoga, so I can have those abilities." By pushing into the edges of your flexibility in an attempt to do that, you can cause damage to your joints.

When you see an incredibly flexible person, it's important to recognize that he or she might be genetically different from you. You wouldn't try to make your eyes blue if they're brown; you don't need to try to make your hips do the super-splits just because someone else's hips can do them. For most of us, the goal of practicing yoga is to be optimally healthy in our own bodies, creating freedom from restriction and pain. The goal is not to impress others with our contortionistic abilities, so let's stop acting like it is.

It may help to close your eyes during stretches, so you can focus on the sensations in your own body without being distracted by what others are doing. It's a human tendency to compare ourselves to others, but your long-term health may depend on resisting this tendency in your yoga classes.

Another thing to be aware of is that people with hypermobility syndromes often experience symptoms of joint damage later in life.

Because their ligaments are so flexible, their joints are relatively unprotected. They're able to force their joints into those extreme positions, but they may be wearing away cartilage as they do so. As with most joint problems, it won't necessarily show up as arthritis for quite a while.

Unfortunately, hypermobile yoga students may be viewed as being "great at yoga" by their teachers, instead of being given instruction on how to protect their joints by holding back on those deep stretches. This is a disservice not only to those students, but to the other students in the room, who may themselves attempt to replicate the hypermobile student's yoga practice. This book will provide you with the foundational understanding you need to protect yourself, whether you're hypermobile or not.

How To Protect Your Connective Tissues

- Avoid deep stretches of ligaments and tendons, as these structures are not able to resume their original shapes after being stretched. Stretching fascia, the covering around muscle tissue, is much safer, because its structure makes it more elastic.
- Perform weight-bearing exercise to strengthen the bones, which continually remodel themselves in response to the forces placed upon them.
- Use care when moving joints, to avoid damaging cartilage; this tissue has a very poor ability to repair itself. The lack of nerve endings in cartilage means that you may not have pain as a warning signal when damage is occurring. Be alert for other warning signs, as discussed in the remainder of this book.
- Be aware of the existence of hypermobility, which may affect you or others in your yoga classes.

Now that we've covered how your connective tissues are structured, it's time to explore how these different tissues are put together to form joints. We'll look at the basic structure of a joint in the next chapter.

This will be the foundation for understanding the specifics of each joint in later chapters.

CHAPTER 2:
JOINTS

A joint is where two bones touch, right?

Nope. Well, ideally not, anyway. Two bones touching is painful.

A joint that's freely movable is called a synovial joint. This is the type of joint that we care about the most in yoga, and if we understand a little bit about the way that synovial joints are structured, we become better able to protect them. So let's take a look at the basic way that joints are put together. In later chapters, I'll illuminate specifics about each joint as we dive in deeper.

On the next page, you'll see a very basic outline of a joint. In the illustration, you'll notice two bones coming toward each other. (Each one is hollow on the inside, as previously discussed.) Notice that the two bones don't actually touch. In general, the bones of each joint have pieces that fit together like a puzzle, but they don't touch; they hover a little bit away from each other. There's no periosteum (that covering of connective tissue around a bone) at a joint. Instead, the ends of the bones are covered in a different tissue: cartilage.

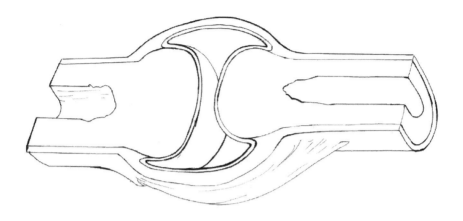

joint structure diagram

This type of cartilage is called articular cartilage; it's a type of hyaline cartilage. The word *hyaline* comes from the Greek word for glass, and hyaline cartilage is, like glass, clear and smooth. In the body, it's slightly bluish in color (but if seen after death, such as in meat, it usually looks more clear or yellowish). It has essentially the same texture as a bouncy ball.

Hyaline cartilage has no blood vessels. That's why it looks blue instead of pink. There are very few cells inside of it; it's almost entirely ground substance and some fibers. Unfortunately, this means that damaged cartilage heals incredibly slowly, if at all.

When excessive forces are placed on the articular cartilage of a joint, such as happens when it's moved in an unsafe way, the cartilage may be worn away. Cartilage has no nerves, and so it often doesn't hurt while it's being damaged. However, once the articular cartilage is gone, then the bones of the joint may begin touching each other. Bones are incredibly innervated; when bone touches bone, it hurts a lot.

When a joint hurts because its cartilage has been worn down, this is called osteoarthritis. Estimates indicate that up to 1 in 3 American adults have osteoarthritis in at least one joint. Unfortunately, once osteoarthritis has occurred, there's not a lot that can be offered to help. Anti-inflammatory medications are often prescribed, but these have many side effects when continued long-term. Some people end up choosing joint replacement surgery, but this is a major surgery and cannot fully replicate the original joint.

Ideally, everyone should try to avoid osteoarthritis. This involves being careful with how we move our joints, not only during yoga practice, but throughout our lives. I hope that understanding each joint will help you to protect yourself both on and off the mat. Of course, I can't promise you that you'll never get osteoarthritis; no one could make a promise like that. However, the knowledge here will empower you to create the best possible chance for your joints to stay healthy.

Synovial Fluid

If cartilage has no blood supply, how do those few cells inside get their nutrients? How do they get rid of their waste products?

The joint space is filled with a fluid called synovial fluid. It's thin, clear, and slippery. Synovial fluid serves several purposes. It lubricates the movements of the joint, and it spreads out the forces the joint experiences so that they don't get concentrated in one small area. It also transports nutrients and waste products to and from the cells inside the cartilage.

Synovial fluid has no pump. It's pushed around in the joint space through movements of the joint itself. This is one reason your joints get stiff when you remain still for a long period. When you get out of the car after a long road trip, your knees and hips feel stiff because they haven't been moving. After you walk around a bit, you get the synovial fluid moving in those joints, and then they feel much better-lubricated.

What keeps the fluid inside the joint? The joint space is defined by the joint capsule, a connective tissue structure surrounding the joint. You can see it around the joint in the illustration above. The capsule's microscopic structure is similar to that of tendon or ligament. On the inner surface of the joint capsule is the thin synovial membrane, which secretes the synovial fluid. The joint capsule is very thick and strong in some joints, and much thinner and weaker in others. As we'll see, joints with a thinner joint capsule require more muscular effort to stabilize them and keep them safe.

The joint capsule has to be loose enough to allow the joint to move. When one side of the joint capsule is taut, the other side is loose, with little folds; when the joint moves to the other end of its range of motion, the folds will be on the opposite side. These folds of capsule have a tendency to stick to each other when the joint is still. When the joint moves, the pieces of the capsule are pulled apart.

If the joint doesn't move, then the stickiness gets worse. The stuck-together parts of the joint capsule are known as adhesions. Once a joint has adhesions, then it can't move anymore. This is why it's important not to fully immobilize a joint if it's at all avoidable. Of course you don't want to force too much movement of a joint that's been injured, but if you completely stop moving it because it hurts, then pretty soon you can't move it due to the formation of adhesions. Adhesions can eventually be broken down, but it may take months of physical therapy.

Ligaments

An extra stabilizing force on the joints is provided by ligaments. Most joints have at least a few, although there's huge variation in how many ligaments each joint has and how strong they are. A joint with fewer ligaments requires muscular effort to stabilize it. For instance, the shoulder, with a thin joint capsule and few ligaments, requires the rotator cuff muscles to be active to keep it safe, particularly if part of the body weight is being borne on the arm.

As discussed in the last chapter, ligaments are made up of type I collagen, arranged in long parallel rows and cross-linked. Stretching the ligament too much breaks the cross-linkages, meaning that the ligament will be permanently longer. With the ligaments too lax to help support the joint, it will become more prone to partially or completely dislocating. It may also move abnormally, and can be pulled into extreme movements that would normally be prevented by the ligaments; either of these can cause wearing down of the articular cartilage. Protecting the ligaments is crucial to keeping a joint stable and healthy for life.

Bursae

The surfaces of bones often have bumps or uneven parts. As muscles contract during movement, their tendons may be drawn across these bumpy surfaces, potentially damaging the tendon. Because of this, it's sometimes necessary for the body to put a cushion over a bony bump, in order to protect a tendon.

This type of a cushion is called a bursa (plural: bursae). It's just a little sac filled with synovial fluid. Certain joints have one or more of them, depending on the structure of the bones and tendons involved.

If a joint is moved in such a way that a bursa is squeezed between two bones, it may lead to bursitis, or inflammation of a bursa. This causes pain, swelling, and stiffness of the joint.

Why Do Joints Crack?

You've almost certainly experienced a "crack" when you move a joint. Why this happens is one of the most common questions I get from students in my workshops and teacher trainings. While the phenomenon isn't completely understood scientifically, there are a few possible reasons behind it.

If a joint cracks each time you move it in a particular way, then it could indicate underlying damage to the joint. Cartilage doesn't heal very well, so when it's been damaged, there's often an uneven spot remaining. When the two cartilage surfaces are rubbed against each other, the damaged spot may rub or catch in such a way that it produces a sound each time it's moved.

If you experience this type of cracking in one of your joints, be mindful of how it feels when it happens. The damaged cartilage is creating abnormal forces moving through the joint, so there's the potential for further cartilage damage and, eventually, osteoarthritis. While I don't recommend immobilizing the joint because of the cracking, you might want to minimize how often you do the movements that cause the sound. If the joint hurts after cracking, then definitely try to minimize it. But a joint that doesn't move enough isn't able to be healthy either, so even if your joint cracks, don't restrict its movement too much.

If a joint cracks the first time you move it, and then doesn't crack at all for a while, you might be experiencing the phenomenon called "creep." When a joint is held in a position that puts abnormal forces on it (for instance, hunching of the mid-back at your desk), the joint slowly slips (or "creeps") into slight misalignment, with the joint surfaces separating from each other. This is basically a very slow partial dislocation, also known as a subluxation.

When you release the abnormal forces and move (for instance, you stand up and stretch your back), the bones slip back into place, which you may hear as a crack or a clunking sound. Now that the joint is back where it belongs, it will move normally, not cracking again (unless you put it back into poor alignment again – for instance, when you sit back down at your desk).

If you have this type of joint cracking, the crack itself isn't a problem. The problem is the joint having been pulled out of alignment in the first place. You wouldn't want to leave the bones of your mid-back slipped out of alignment with each other, because that could cause significant problems with those joints over time; putting them back into place is much healthier for them. So don't avoid the cracking.

However, if you can, address the postural issue that led to the joints creeping in the first place. For instance, if your mid-back cracks every time you get up from your chair at work, then you might want to consider getting a different chair, or working on your posture to better support your back. Don't try to stop it from cracking; try to stop it from needing to crack.

These are only two possible reasons for joints to crack. There are other possibilities, although research hasn't been definitive on what causes it in every case. As far as most research shows, it appears that cracking joints doesn't damage them. So, while I wouldn't advise you to crack your joints excessively, if some of your joints crack, it's probably not something to worry about. If there's pain or discomfort with the cracking, then talk to your doctor about it.

Fibrous and Cartilaginous Joints

Synovial joints are the most important joints to know about, both in yoga practice and in daily life, because they're the ones that move most freely. However, there are two other types of joints in the body.

Fibrous joints are joints that don't move at all. The two bones are held tightly together by connective tissue. For example, your skull is made up of several different bones; once your head is no longer growing, the joints between them become fibrous joints called sutures, with essentially no ability to move relative to one another.

Cartilaginous joints have a small ability to move. At these joints, a disc of fibrocartilage (a stiffer form of cartilage) sits between the two bones. The disc is firmly attached to each bone, but the bones have some ability to move relative to each other by squishing, stretching, and twisting the disc. Examples include the joints between the main parts of the vertebrae of the spine, and the pubic symphysis, where the two halves of the pelvis come together.

Cartilaginous joints are not as vulnerable as synovial joints, but they're not completely immune to damage, either. Damage to the discs is possible, so knowing about these joints can be helpful in ensuring that the body stays safe during movement; we'll discuss them in more detail in later chapters.

The Movement of Joints

Now that you understand how a joint is constructed, the next step is to explore the muscles that move the joints. In the next chapter, we'll look at the muscles, the fascia, and how the forces that move your body are produced. This will be helpful in learning how to protect your muscles, fascia, and tendons from injury.

CHAPTER 3:
MUSCLES

Although we use our muscles throughout each day, most people aren't familiar with them on the deepest levels. How are they constructed? How can we ensure that we both use them appropriately, and protect them from harm?

To begin our exploration, let's zoom way, way in, to look at a muscle on the microscopic level.

Sarcomeres

A sarcomere is the basic contractile unit of a muscle: the "brick" of a muscle, so to speak.

two sarcomeres

Within each sarcomere, long proteins are interleaved with each other. When it's signaled to contract, one of the proteins (actin) binds to the other (myosin), ratcheting itself along to pull the two sides of the sarcomere closer together. At a basic level, that's all a muscle can do: bring one end of itself closer to the other end (i.e., get shorter).

The sarcomeres are arranged in long parallel strands called myofibrils. When the muscle contracts, lots of sarcomeres shorten together, bringing the ends of the muscle closer to each other.

When a muscle gets stronger, it doesn't create extra muscle cells; it adds more sarcomeres to the existing muscle cells. (It can also do other things that make it more efficient, such as adding more of the machinery that creates energy for muscle contraction, and enhancing its connection to the nervous system.) Research indicates that the body doesn't create any new muscle cells past infancy, but instead it invests in growing and repairing the cells that it has in order to make them stronger.

Some research suggests that if a muscle is just worked out, then sarcomeres will be added primarily in the center of the muscle, thus making the muscle appear larger. However, if a muscle is worked out and then stretched, then sarcomeres are more likely to be added evenly across the muscle. This could explain why yoga practitioners, dancers, and gymnasts get strong, but rarely look large, while weightlifters get large muscles. The research on this is far from definitive, but it's an intriguing idea.

Muscle Fibers

The muscles that you control voluntarily are called your skeletal muscles. There are other types of muscle, including cardiac muscle (in your heart) and smooth muscle (in your other organs), but you can't exercise direct voluntary control over these. Yoga does have several benefits to these types of muscle, but skeletal muscle is the type we're most concerned about when discussing yoga safety, so we'll focus on it here.

Skeletal muscle cells are formed by the fusion of many smaller cells during embryological life. Each muscle cell is very large and has many nuclei (the part of a cell that houses its genetic material). In essence, the small pre-muscle cells fuse into a larger organization, to enhance their ability to accomplish their work in the world. The resulting mega-cell is called a muscle fiber.

A skeletal muscle is made up of many muscle fibers, all arranged in parallel. All of the muscle fibers pull in the same direction, working together to create a muscle contraction.

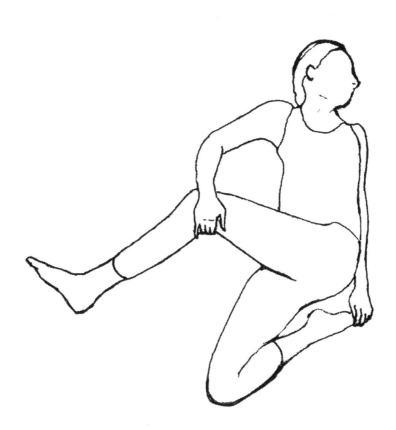

supine spinal twist with bottom knee bent

When the muscle is placed in a shortened position, it tends to start contracting involuntarily – meaning that you get a muscle cramp. This comes up sometimes in yoga. For instance, if you're in a supine spinal twist, and you decide to deepen it by bending the bottom knee and holding the foot with your hand, then the hamstrings of your bottom leg are in a shortened position and may begin cramping.

There's nothing dangerous about these cramps, and they're usually easily relieved by lengthening the muscle again. However, they're quite uncomfortable, and most people prefer to avoid them if possible.

Fascia

Every muscle has fascia (FASH-uh), or connective tissue, surrounding it. There are three layers of fascia. The first layer surrounds each muscle fiber itself; the enormously large, multinucleated muscle cell is wrapped in this thin layer of fascia, known as the endomysium (en-doh-MIH-zee-um).

The next layer, called perimysium (pair-ah-MIH-zee-um), wraps several muscle fibers together into a bundle called a fascicle (FAS-ih-cull). These are the "strings" you might have seen in a piece of meat. In some of your muscles, you might be able to feel them below the surface of your skin, especially in a muscle that's fairly large (for instance, you've been weight-training it).

Finally, a layer of fascia surrounds the whole muscle. It binds together all of the fascicles, along with blood vessels and nerves. This is the epimysium (ep-ih-MIH-zee-um).

When you stretch a muscle, you always stretch its fascia, and vice versa. The two are intimately connected. It's not possible to stretch something without stretching the covering around it. So although some forms of yoga may claim to be stretching fascia rather than muscles, this isn't really possible. You can't stretch fascia without stretching muscles. You also can't stretch muscles without stretching fascia.

At the ends of the muscle, the fascia becomes a tendon. There's no clear boundary here; rather, the structure of fascia slowly fades into the structure of tendon. This zone is called the myotendinous junction.

Because the myotendinous junction is a transition zone, it's a bit disorganized at the microscopic level. As a result, this is the most vulnerable part of the muscle. If a muscle is going to tear, this is the most likely place for it to happen. That's why it's important to protect this part of the muscle.

The tendon may be short or long, depending on the muscle. Once it reaches the target bone, the tendon becomes periosteum. Again, there's not a clear boundary between the two structures; it's more of a gradual transition. However, because the structures of tendon and periosteum are much more similar at the microscopic level than are tendon and fascia, there's less disorganization in the transition zone between them, and the junction of tendon and bone is less vulnerable to damage than is the myotendinous junction.

Recall that bones respond to the forces placed on them. At the point of attachment of a tendon, the bone experiences significant force in a concentrated way. Bones respond by forming bumps or ridges wherever tendons are attached. The larger the muscle, the larger the force; therefore, the larger the bony bump that will result. For instance, your ischial tuberosities (or "sit bones") are bony bumps under your pelvis; they're large because the powerful hamstrings attach there. There's a bump on the front of your shin at the top of the tibia where the quadriceps tendon attaches. These types of structures can be found throughout the body; anywhere a bone has a big bump, you know that the tendon of a large muscle attaches there.

Proprioception

Close your eyes, then describe the position of your legs.

Without looking at your legs, you know where each part is, relative to other parts and in space. This sense, which (like all of our senses) we usually take for granted, is called proprioception – literally, the sensing of oneself.

Like most of our senses, proprioception is more sensitive to changes than to a constant stimulus. If you've been completely still for a period, you might feel like you've partially lost the sense of the position of your body. Even the tiniest movement can then bring your proprioceptive sense flooding back. You may have experienced this phenomenon during a particularly deep savasana (the rest pose at the end of yoga), when you were completely still for several minutes. When it was time to come out, a small movement of a finger can bring back a sudden sense of having a body.

There are two main proprioceptive organs that you should be aware of as a yoga practitioner: muscle spindles and Golgi tendon organs. Both have relevance to the safety and the effectiveness of your yoga practice.

Muscle spindles are embedded throughout each muscle, positioned between the muscle fibers. Their function is to detect the stretch of the muscle. When a muscle stretches very quickly or too deeply, the muscle spindles trigger a reflex contraction of that muscle, to protect it from a possible tear. Yoga practitioners experience this as a feeling of resistance, as though the body is resisting the stretch – which it is.

The muscle spindle will slow its firing after a muscle has been at a given length for about a minute or so. You may have had the experience of being in a pose for several breaths, and then you felt a sudden "melting," a feeling of sinking a little deeper into the pose. This was the point where your muscle spindles quieted down.

One of the things that happens as you "get more flexible" is that you train your muscle spindles to fire less. They tolerate a longer muscle length before they trigger a contraction that stops any deepening. Interestingly, many exercise scientists believe that this is exclusively what happens as you stretch: the structure of the muscle doesn't get any longer, but the nervous system learns to tolerate a longer length. There is some debate on this, but the muscle spindle is definitely an important determinant of your flexibility.

If you continue to force a deeper stretch while the muscle is contracting and resisting that stretch, you're likely to get injured. The muscle itself can't get any longer while it's contracting, so the stretch will be concentrated at vulnerable zones like the myotendinous junction. The muscle tissue itself may also be torn, as some sarcomeres generally contract more strongly than others, and those that are contracting less may be torn apart. Although you get more flexible by teaching your nervous system to tolerate a longer muscle length, you can't do this all at once. Instead, once you feel that contraction start, back off just a bit and hold the stretch for several long breaths. It's likely that the muscle will release as the muscle spindles quiet down.

The Golgi tendon organ is embedded within each tendon near the myotendinous junction, that most vulnerable part of the muscle-tendon complex, and is also stimulated by stretching. When it detects a fast or deep stretch of the tendon, the Golgi tendon organ triggers a reflex relaxation of the muscle. This protects the myotendinous junction from damage by releasing some of the tension on the tendon. Using this muscle relaxation to deepen a stretch may result in tearing the myotendinous junction, which can take a long time to heal.

Muscle Quivering

I have yoga students ask me about quivering muscles pretty regularly. Is it okay if a muscle starts shaking when you're in a pose? Does it mean that you should come out of the pose?

First of all, let's consider what actually happens during a muscle contraction. It's not as simple as all of the muscle fibers within the muscle contracting at once. Each muscle fiber can contract for only a certain length of time before it starts to fatigue. This is determined by the availability of energy in the body (your blood sugar) as well as characteristics of the muscle fiber itself. When the muscle fiber gets tired, it will not be able to contract, even when the nervous system is telling it to.

Also, a given muscle fiber is either contracting or relaxed. There's no partial contraction of a muscle cell; it's just an on/off switch. Yet you know that you can produce a huge range of contractions of a muscle, from a very gentle contraction to a very strong one. How is your body accomplishing this?

A single motor nerve ending makes contact with a few muscle fibers within a muscle. The grouping is called a *motor unit*. When the nerve fires, all of those fibers will contract together. How many muscle cells are in a motor unit depends on the muscle. The finer the control needed, the smaller the motor units – meaning that there are fewer muscle fibers controlled by each nerve, and therefore more nerve endings in that particular muscle. With more nerve endings, each controlling only a few muscle fibers, the brain is able to more precisely control the movements of the muscle.

The motor units in the muscles that control your hand and fingers, which require very fine control, are very small, with a large proportion of your total motor neurons devoted to these muscles. For the muscles of your back, each motor unit is much larger, containing many more muscle fibers, and the precision of your control over these muscles is correspondingly reduced.

When a muscle contracts, the brain does not simply activate all of the motor units in the muscle. In fact, even at a maximal contraction of the muscle, all of the motor units aren't activated; only about a third of them are active at any point in time. During a prolonged contraction of the muscle, the brain rotates through the motor units seamlessly, allowing each to contract for a period and then rest for a period, so that the contraction can be maintained. You usually won't notice this switching between different motor units.

Once some of the muscle fibers start to become fatigued, however, this rotation pattern becomes obvious. As the brain rotates through the fibers, some of them are too tired to produce a contraction, while others are still able to contract. This shows up as a quivering or shaking in the muscle. Basically, a shaking muscle is a fatigued muscle.

When you experience this type of shaking, it doesn't mean that you have to come out of the pose right away. You're at your limit of strength, and if you stay in the pose, you're going to be sore tomorrow. I wouldn't recommend pushing through that shaking indefinitely, but if you spend a little longer in the pose, you won't cause any real harm. At the end of a vigorous yoga practice, many practitioners notice shaking of some of their muscles. (This shaking is worse when your blood sugar is low, because the muscle fibers fatigue faster when deprived of fuel. So if you get a lot of shaking during yoga, you might want to consider eating a little more during the meal prior to class, or even drinking some juice or a smoothie fifteen minutes before class, to fuel up. I know what some will say – eating within two hours of class is yoga heresy!)

Fatigue isn't the only reason for a muscle to shake. It also happens when the muscle spindles are detect a stretch that's too deep, and attempt to contract the muscle to protect it, but can't do so effectively. While the muscle is under a stretch, it's at a mechanical disadvantage, and may not be able to generate much power. However, when it feels threatened, it will still try. This overly stretched muscle will quiver as it tries to generate enough force to make itself shorter.

If this is the reason your muscle is quivering, then you need to come out of the pose right away. Your muscle is trying to tell you that it can't handle what you're doing to it, and it's about to be harmed. You definitely shouldn't keep stretching at this point.

So how can you tell the difference between these two reasons for a quivering muscle? You pay attention to exactly which muscle is quivering.

For example, let's say that you're doing a hamstring stretch, lying on your back with your foot up toward the ceiling (as shown in the illustration on the next page). Your knee is straight, so your quads are working to extend the knee. You notice your leg quivering.

If your quads are quivering, then you're safe. It's just that the quads are working hard to keep your knee straight against gravity (which would love to pull that foot downward), and they're getting tired. You can stay in the pose a little longer if you'd like, although you'd certainly be justified in deciding that you've had enough for that day and coming out of the pose to rest the leg.

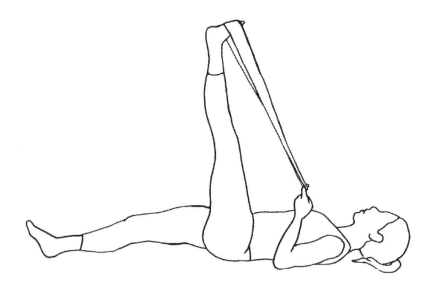

supine hamstring stretch

However, if your hamstrings are quivering, then you need to release the tension on them immediately. By quivering while being stretched, they're indicating that the stretch is too deep. Bend your knee slightly, or lower your straight leg toward the ground. Otherwise, you may end up tearing your hamstring, which is not fun.

When a working muscle is quivering, it's just working hard. When a stretching muscle is quivering, it's in a potential danger zone.

Reciprocal Inhibition

Another useful tidbit about the control of muscles by the nervous system is the fact that antagonist muscles inhibit each other via reflex arcs.

Antagonist muscles are muscles that perform opposite actions. For instance, the quadriceps extend (straighten) the knee, while the hamstrings flex (bend) the knee; these are antagonist muscles.

When a muscle contracts, the contraction of its antagonist is inhibited. In other words, when the quads contract, the hamstrings relax. This happens through a reflex at the spinal cord level, so it's not under your conscious control. This phenomenon is called reciprocal inhibition.

It is possible to co-contract antagonist muscles, by consciously sending the impulse to contract to both of the muscles at the same time. However, neither muscle will be able to achieve maximal contraction, because of the mutual reciprocal inhibition.

You can use reciprocal inhibition to your advantage. Let's say that you want to stretch your hamstrings in a seated forward fold.

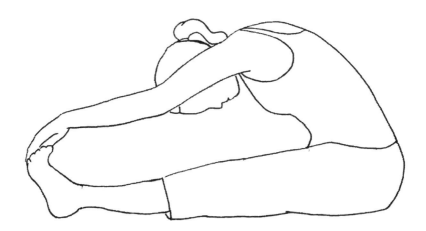

seated forward fold (paschimottanasana)

By contracting your quads (the most useful cues for this are "lift your kneecaps" or "straighten your knees"), you'll achieve reflex inhibition of the hamstrings, so that they don't resist the stretch. In this case, the relaxation of the hamstrings could also protect the low back. (To understand how the hamstrings and the low back are linked, see the Low Back chapter.) Use caution with this; if you "take up the slack" produced by reciprocal inhibition by maximally deepening the stretch, and then you relax the quads a bit, the hamstrings may start contracting to protect themselves, and damage could occur. If you use reciprocal inhibition, maintain it throughout the stretch, and stay away from the absolute edge of your range.

How to Protect Your Muscles

- When a muscle is quivering while stretching, you should immediately release the stretch, to avoid damage.
- When a muscle is quivering while contracting, the muscle is fatigued, but continuing to use it won't cause serious damage.
- If a muscle tightens in response to a stretch, don't go any deeper, to protect the muscle and tendon from tearing. If you stay in the stretch for several long breaths, the resistance may release.
- You can use reciprocal inhibition to relax a muscle that's being stretched, but use caution so that you don't hurt yourself.

Armed with knowledge about the body and how it works, it's time to look at the general guidelines for keeping the body safe. After we get a general sense of what this looks like, then we'll explore specific parts of the body in the later sections of this book. The concepts presented in the next chapter will be referenced again and again throughout the remaining sections of this book.

If you remember only one chapter from this book, the next one should be it!

CHAPTER 4:
SAFE VS. UNSAFE SENSATIONS

This chapter is the core of the book. I've lost count of how many times students have told me what they're feeling in a pose and asked, "Is that okay?" When you start a yoga practice, it can seem difficult just to untangle what you're actually feeling, let alone to interpret what it means. Even after practicing for years, many students don't really know the meanings all of their bodily sensations.

Yoga teachers may tell students in class, "Listen to your body." While this is great advice, it can be hard follow it if you're not sure what various sensations mean. Some meanings are obvious, such as that sharp pain in a joint indicates that you're hurting yourself. But what about squeezing in a joint? What about a deep stretch near a joint? How do you know what's safe and what's not?

In this chapter, I'll present the basic information that will allow you to protect yourself whenever you practice yoga. This will give you a foundation that will allow you to decode the sensations you feel in various poses. In the remainder of the book, we'll dive into specific joints and areas of the body, exploring these concepts in more detail.

What's Safe and What's Not?

Unfortunately, in many yoga classes, there's little information about safety. Many yoga traditions seem to believe that the most "advanced" yogis are the ones who can go deepest into a pose, so the whole goal of these classes is to go as deep as possible, and to force your body to develop additional flexibility.

There may be instructions about alignment in many classes. It may seem like the alignment instructions are there to protect your body. However, keep in mind the environment in which these alignments were developed. For the most part, the ancient yogis were supremely unconcerned with protecting the body; their aim was to transcend it. In some traditions, the goal was to come into an uncomfortable pose and then hold it as long as possible, practicing stilling the mind and remaining serene despite the discomfort. The long-term consequences of doing this were generally not considered.

While serenity is a noble goal, I don't believe that it's necessary to damage the body to achieve that. I see a certain thread of this particular ancient tradition running through much yoga today, however, with the instructions to take each pose to its very edge and then breathe there, staying calm even though it hurts. "Breathe into the discomfort," or some variation of that, is a common instruction in many modern yoga classes. Just be aware that this idea is out there, and that you may even have inherited some of it from your own teachers.

In the middle of the 20th century, a new attempt was made to create alignment in yoga, mainly through the Iyengar tradition. Some of the resulting alignment instructions do indeed make poses safer; for example, keeping the knee directly over the middle of the foot in a lunge protects the cartilage of the kneecap.

However, other alignment instructions have nothing to do with safety. Many of them make a pose more aesthetically-pleasing. Others make a pose harder, so that you get stronger. And there are many alignment instructions with an unclear origin.

The yoga masters who created the pose alignments we still follow today were, for the most part, not educated about biomechanics. None had studied the subject deeply in an academic setting. They also lacked the benefit of scientific studies of large populations, and of technology that could visualize the inside of a living body, both of which we're fortunate to have today. They knew incredible amounts about their own bodies. But that's it. So don't assume that by following their instructions, you're keeping yourself safe.

Much of what we teach as yoga teachers has simply been handed down to us, and is coming through us without necessarily being filtered through our own critical thinking. (To be fair, the same is true in most professions.) Most teachers are taught the "correct" alignments of a pose in training, and then parrot that information to their students, believing that they're serving them well. Very few teachers acquire the understanding necessary to feel confident in altering the instructions they were taught.

My goal with this book is to help you understand the body well enough to know which alignment instructions are which, so that you're empowered to keep your body safe whenever you take a yoga class or practice on your own, and to keep your students safe if you're a yoga teacher.

Tension Versus Compression

The Yin Yoga system has developed the idea of tension and compression to explain safe and unsafe sensations in a pose. While this is a useful framework, I believe it's a little limited; I'll be expanding on it to help you really understand which sensations are okay and which are potentially dangerous.

To use the tension and compression system, you go into a pose until you hit some kind of an edge – not necessarily pain, but a feeling that you're at the limit of your flexibility. Then you ask yourself, what do I feel? What's stopping me from going further into this pose? The answer might be tension – tightness, pulling, stretching. Or it might be compression – pinching, squeezing, a feeling of not having space in a joint. Tension is sometimes okay, while compression never is. Let's explore them both.

Tension

Let's say you're going into a forward bend. At some point, you stop, because you feel deep stretching along the backs of your legs. This could indicate stretching of one of a number of different structures, so you need to determine where you're feeling that sensation to decide whether it means you should back out of the pose a bit.

If you're feeling the stretch all along the back of your leg, then it's a result of stretching the muscle (and fascia). This is a safe sensation. While it doesn't have to feel perfectly comfortable, since new sensations often feel a little strange, it also shouldn't feel painful. If the stretch feels painful, then you're at risk for tearing the muscle that you're stretching, so you should back out of the pose a little bit. As long as the stretch isn't too deep, then there's no problem with stretching muscle tissue and fascia, because both of them are extensible; they won't be permanently lengthened in an unsafe way. Most people find stretching (in the safe range) to be quite pleasant, and many even crave it.

However, if you're feeling the stretch near a joint or a bone, then you're in a danger zone. You may be feeling the tendon of a muscle being stretched; for example, in the forward bend, you could feel that sensation close to your sit bones or behind your knee (where the hamstring tendons are). This is not a safe sensation, for a few reasons. Because tendons can't be stretched very much without causing permanent lengthening, it's not a good idea to be stretching tendons. Also, the myotendinous junction (where the muscle meets the tendon) is a very vulnerable spot. If the muscle is going to tear, that's where it's likely to happen. So if you're feeling a stretch in the region of the tendon, back out of the pose. You want the stretch to be all along the muscle, not concentrated in its ends.

A stretch near a joint could also indicate the stretching of ligaments or the joint capsule. These structures aren't elastic and won't bounce back if stretched. If the ligaments or joint capsule become lengthened, they will no longer be able to fulfill their role of keeping the joint stable. This is likely to lead to abnormal movement patterns, which then wear down the cartilage and eventually lead to osteoarthritis. It also makes the joint vulnerable to being dislocated.

It's extremely important not to stretch out your ligaments and joint capsules if you want to keep your joints healthy. If you feel a stretch near a joint, adjust or back out of the stretch, until you're feeling it in muscle instead of joint.

Compression

The other sensation that can limit the depth you achieve in a pose is compression. It's often described as a pinching or squeezing in a joint, or as just "having no space" in that joint.

When you feel compression in a joint, that indicates that two bones in the joint are very close together, and the cartilage is being squeezed. (Because cartilage isn't well-innervated, you're not necessarily feeling the cartilage itself, but the tissues around it being squeezed.) This is the absolute edge of your ability to safely perform a pose. If you try to go deeper, you may be able to do so, but not without a cost. By putting excessive pressure on the articular surfaces, you'll wear away the cartilage, which is likely to lead to osteoarthritis.

If you stay in a pose despite a feeling of compression, you'll often come out of the pose with an ache in the joint, caused by the tissues around the cartilage being squeezed. You may be able to "release the stretch" with some movement, and the pain will go away. However, remember that cartilage has very few nerves. Even though your joint no longer hurts, there may have been significant damage to the cartilage.

Range of Motion

Straighten your elbow all the way.

That's easy for most people; you feel an obvious end-point to the movement. You aren't saying to yourself, "If only my bicep were more flexible, I could straighten my elbow much farther! I'm so tight!" You can tell that the limit on your elbow extension is imposed by the shape of your bones.

All joints have points like this, but it's not always as obvious to us. When you come to a similar point in your hip, you may not be aware that you've reached an end-point imposed by the shape of the bones. You may think, "I'm so tight! I need to stretch more, so I can go deeper into this pose!" You may be able to force a greater range of motion, but this will cause damage.

I find it extremely unfortunate that there seems to be very little understanding of this idea among yoga teachers. I frequently hear students being told to "work on their flexibility," when what they describe is a feeling of compression that indicates that they've gone as far into the pose as they safely can go.

The feeling of compression in a joint is what tells you that you've reached the natural endpoint of your range of motion for that joint. Trying to force it to go further is not a good idea. When you feel squeezing inside a joint, think of it like your elbow during that straightening exercise, and recognize that you've reached your natural flexibility limit. This could even be thought of as an opportunity to celebrate; you've released your muscle tension enough to allow you to reach the limits of your joint's range of motion, and your movements are now free.

Tingling

In some cases, a pose may lead to sensations far from the affected joints. For instance, a deep shoulder stretch could lead to tingling in the fingers. This is a warning sign of nerve damage.

When a nerve is under duress (either being pinched or excessively stretched), a predictable sequence of symptoms occurs. First, there's tingling. This results from the sensory nerves sending abnormal signals. You've probably experienced this type of tingling when you "bumped your funny bone," which compresses the ulnar nerve of the forearm and hand in its least protected spot at the elbow. (We'll come back to the ulnar nerve in Chapter 9.)

If the compression or stretch of the nerve persists for a period of time, the tingling progresses to numbness. The sensory nerve cells have lost their ability to signal. Later, the motor nerve cells begin to be affected as well, leading to weakness in the area. (Because the motor nerve cells are larger than the sensory ones, it takes longer for them to show the effects.)

The old-school traditional instructions were often to sit through the tingling because it would go away. I've still heard this said; if your feet are tingling when you sit in lotus, don't worry, just stay through the discomfort and it'll go away soon.

It will go away – when it progresses to numbness. If you keep doing it, then you'll get weakness. That causes disability. Which is not the same as enlightenment.

When tingling occurs, the nervous system is being damaged, and it's crucial to take this warning seriously. While peripheral nerves themselves can regenerate to some degree (because they're just long projections from nerve cells located in or near the spinal cord), when nerve damage progresses, the nerve cells themselves start to die. It's long been thought that nerve cells that die are never replaced, and while recent research indicates that this might not be completely true, it's still very close to the truth. For the most part, nerve cells that die are lost forever. If you ignore signals that your nerves are in danger, the damage may be permanent.

The adjustment that's needed to release the tingling and protect the nerve is usually not huge. For instance, someone whose foot is tingling because they're sitting on their sciatic nerve may find that an inch or two of adjustment in how the legs are positioned fixes the problem. You may have to shift around for a while to find what works for your body. This effort is well-spent.

How To Protect Yourself in Yoga

- Keep the sensation of stretching all along the length of a muscle. If you feel a stretch near a joint, back out a bit, to protect the tendon and myotendinous junction.
- Don't allow stretching to be painful, to protect the muscle and associated connective tissue structures from tearing.
- If you feel compression (pinching, squeezing) in a joint, back out of the stretch a bit, to avoid damage to the articular cartilage.
- If you feel tingling, adjust the pose so that you don't feel it anymore, to protect your nerve cells.

Now that you have a set of general guidelines for determining which sensations are safe and which aren't, let's start to dive into specific parts of the body to apply these ideas in a more concrete way. We'll start with the core of the body, exploring the spine. If you've ever had back pain, this next chapter is for you.

SECTION 2:
THE SPINE

Traditional yoga theory puts a lot of emphasis on the spine. The spine is considered the channel through which energy flows, connecting the various energy centers of the body. Yoga practitioners know the spine is key to health, but don't necessarily understand its structure and how to protect it during yoga. Unfortunately, potentially dangerous movements of the spine are encouraged in many yoga traditions.

In this section, we'll explore the physical structure of the spine. First, we'll look at the spine in general. This includes consideration of posture, and the various ways that the spine can move. Next, we'll explore two regions that give many people trouble: the neck and the low back. Stiffness and discomfort in these regions is very common in modern society. The neck requires extra protection, as it contains structures that can lead to devastating consequences when injured.

Let's start with an overview of the spine.

CHAPTER 5:
POSTURE

The health of the back is a major concern for most people who begin a yoga practice. In the modern world, our physical environment doesn't tend to support the health of the spine. As a result, many people struggle with back pain and stiffness.

For example, consider your car, in which (if you're like most people) you spend a significant amount of time nearly every day. Cars aren't designed to drive; they're designed to crash. The driver's seat of a car curves toward the back of the car. During a crash, the force of the impact will be absorbed slowly, as the driver is thrown back into that curved seat, rather than all at once (as it would be if the seat were straight). That helps to protect your spine from being damaged in the crash. Unfortunately, it also forces you to hunch your back as you drive, which tends to make your back sore and stiff.

That's far from the only example. Many people spend time on a couch or in a cushy armchair daily, which promotes hunching of the back. We bend forward to look at our smartphones and tablets. Many carry heavy bags regularly; even children are often asked to carry heavy backpacks, promoting hunching. In all of these ways and more, our physical environment works against our spinal health.

Many people come to yoga to help relieve their back pain, and some studies have shown that it does have an effect. However, when extreme spinal movements are included in a yoga practice, it can become damaging rather than healing.

To protect the back, we need to understand its structure. Let's start with the "bricks" that make up the spinal column: the vertebrae.

Vertebrae

The spinal column is made up of many small bones stacked on top of each other. Each bone is called a vertebra (because it's Latin, the plural is vertebrae). There are 24 separate vertebrae in the spine, plus the sacrum and coccyx, which are created by the fusion of several vertebrae each.

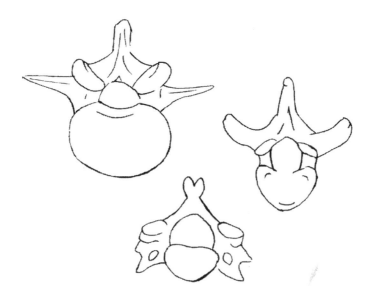

vertebrae: lumbar at upper left, thoracic at upper right, cervical at bottom

The vertebrae share a common basic structure, with various modifications in different parts of the spine. In this illustration, you see three different vertebrae; soon, we'll be exploring the sections of the spine and why they're different.

The main weight-bearing portion is the body of the vertebra, a thick cylinder of bone. In the illustration above, the bodies of the vertebrae look like circles, as they're being viewed from above; you can see the vertebral body at the bottom of each image. The vertebral bodies become larger as you travel down the spine, since the lower parts need to bear more body weight. These are stacked up on each other (separated by discs of cartilage) to form the column through which the forces of body weight are primarily transferred. The vertebral bodies form the front of the spine, meaning that it's the part inside of your body. That means you can't feel your vertebral bodies from the outside.

The spinal cord itself is located behind the bodies of the vertebrae, in the spinal canal. In the illustration, you can see a space that's roughly circular located behind the vertebral bodies; imagine these spaces stacked on top of each other to form a long tube. Inside of this bony tube is the spinal cord, the all-important structure that all of the bone is there to protect, floating in a cushion of cerebrospinal fluid.

Behind that (at the top of each image) is the spinous process, which can be felt on your back as a series of bony bumps (your "dinosaur spikes"). To the sides are the transverse processes, which are usually difficult to feel from the outside because they're covered by muscle. The spinous and transverse processes are sites for the attachment of muscles that move the spine.

Spinal Nerves

The spinal cord is part of the central nervous system, and creates two-way communication between the brain and the body. Unfortunately, because it's made up of nerve cells, its ability to regenerate when injured is very limited. When the spinal cord is damaged, the part of the body below the injury becomes both numb and paralyzed, because it's no longer able to communicate with the brain. This is why the protection of the spinal cord is crucial.

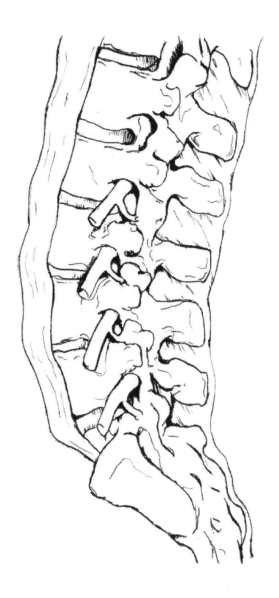

lumbar spine with spinal nerves

The spinal cord sends out many spinal nerves to the body. Each vertebra has a small notch on the bottom on each side, and another on the top. When stacked on top of each other, there's a little hole, called a foramen (plural: foramina), between each pair. Through this hole, a nerve passes, containing a wealth of information flowing both ways. It's important to protect these nerves. If they're overly stretched or compressed, their transmissions are interrupted; eventually, the damage becomes permanent. This was discussed more fully in Chapter 4.

In the illustration on the previous page, you can see two empty vertebral foramina at the top, and four spinal nerves passing through their foramina below that. Toward the left of the illustration are the vertebral bodies; toward the right are the spinous processes.

Ligaments

The spine is supported by ligaments, which help to hold the vertebrae in alignment with each other. The longitudinal ligaments run all the way up and down both the front (anterior) and back (posterior) of the vertebral column, holding the bodies of the vertebrae in alignment with each other. The anterior longitudinal ligament can be seen in the illustration above, on the left of the image, running along the vertebral bodies. Other ligaments connect the spinous and transverse processes of adjacent vertebrae; if you look at the right of the same illustration, you'll see some of these ligaments attached to the spinous processes. These connective tissues help to keep the vertebrae from slipping off of each other.

Extremely deep movements of the spine can stretch out these ligaments, leading to instability. For example, plow pose causes extremely deep flexion of the neck; this can stretch out the spinal ligaments. Deep twisting can also cause excessive stretching of these ligaments.

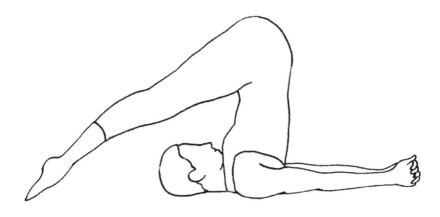

plow pose

Like all ligaments, the ligaments of the spine are important in keeping the joints stable. They prevent the vertebrae from slipping off of each other. If they're stretched too far, the vertebrae will become significantly more prone to subluxation, where they slip out of alignment when placed in a posture that's not ideal (which, for most people, happens pretty often). Because they're ligaments, once they're stretched, their ability to bounce back after a deep stretch is very limited (as discussed in Chapter 1). The tendency of yogis to go into very deep twists and other extreme spinal positions is potentially worrisome for this reason.

If your ligaments become too stretched out, you might notice an increase in your back cracking, as your vertebrae begin to slip off of each other more often. As discussed in Chapter 4, the crack occurs when you bring them back into alignment as you move, so don't avoid the crack; do your best to avoid the need for the crack. If you notice this happening, be aware that it could be your body's warning sign that you've been moving your spine too deeply, and you might want to consider not pushing yourself as far in these poses.

Natural Curves

The spine needs to be able to absorb the forces placed on it when you walk, run, or jump. A straight, rigid column would likely end up breaking at some point (imagine a stick that you pounded on the ground repeatedly every day; it wouldn't last long). Instead of being a straight column, the spine has several natural curves. This gives it a springiness, so it can bend slightly to absorb force. You can see the curves in the illustration below.

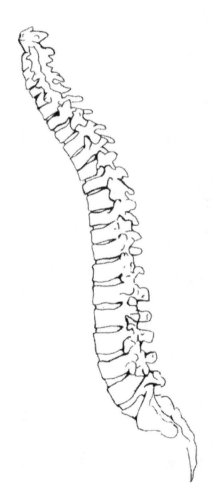

the whole spine

The neck region is called the cervical spine; it has 7 vertebrae. The cervical spine curves toward the front of the body when you're standing up straight (with a neutral spine). The mid-back is called the thoracic spine, has 12 vertebrae, and curves backward at rest. The low back, or lumbar region, has 5 vertebrae and a forward curve. The last five vertebrae are fused together to make a single bone called the sacrum, which again curves backward. You can feel these curves if you run your fingers along your back or look in a mirror while standing up straight. (For those of you who find "standing up straight" to be a challenge, in a few sections, I'll present a method for checking your posture against the wall.)

To refer to a specific vertebra, a letter and a number are used. The letter refers to the spinal region: C for cervical, T for thoracic, L for lumbar, S for sacral. The numbers start with 1 at the top and continue downward. So C1 is the top vertebra, T4 is the fourth one down in the thoracic spine, and L5 is the bottom vertebra of the lumbar spine. (S1 through S5 are fused into one bone; however, the term "S1" is still used to denote the top of the sacrum.)

Interestingly, you aren't born with all of your spinal curves. Only the thoracic and sacral curves are present at birth; these are called the "primary curves" for this reason, and it's no coincidence that child's pose recreates this position. When a baby learns to hold its head up, the cervical curve begins to form. When the toddler learns to walk upright, that's when the lumbar curve starts to take shape. At least, that's the traditional teaching, although some research suggests a very rudimentary lumbar curve may exist earlier; still, the full curve doesn't form until the baby walks. (Dogs, cats, and other animals that walk on four legs don't have lumbar curves.)

The curves serve a purpose; you don't want to get rid of them. As mentioned earlier, the curves allow your spine to absorb the force of walking in a healthy way; without them, your spine would be at increased risk of degeneration. However, you also don't want to exaggerate the curves.

For example, many people find their thoracic spines curved too far backward – i.e., they're "hunching." This excessive thoracic curve may lead to back pain and stiffness. Once they become aware of this problem, many people overcompensate by thrusting the chest forward, attempting to completely remove the thoracic curve; this is also not particularly healthy for the spine.

Discs

The bodies of the vertebrae aren't stacked directly on top of each other, nor are they covered in articular cartilage like most joints. Instead, they form cartilaginous joints. Between the bodies of each pair of vertebrae is an intervertebral disc. The discs are structured somewhat like a jelly donut. Inside, there's a jelly-like substance called the nucleus pulposus; wrapped around it, in concentric circles, are multiple layers of connective tissue. These are made of fibrocartilage, which is somewhere between a tendon and cartilage in structure. (Think of cartilage with a lot of collagen in it.)

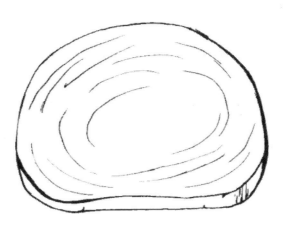

an intervertebral disc

The discs are attached to the bodies of the vertebrae above and below them. That prevents the discs from slipping out from between the vertebrae, which is important in protecting the spinal cord. It also constrains the movements between the vertebral bodies. When the vertebrae move relative to each other, they don't slide off the discs; rather, they squish the discs. For example, when you forward bend, the front sides of the vertebrae move closer together, and the front part of the disc is squished. This pushes the central jelly-like substance towards the back.

If the pressure on the disc is too great, then the nucleus pulposus will break through the stronger layers surrounding it. If it breaks through some of the layers, then the disc becomes a bulging disc. If it breaks all the way through, that's a herniated disc.

The longitudinal ligaments, which run up and down the front and back of the bodies of the vertebrae, help to protect the discs and prevent herniation. They provide a force that resists the poking out of the jelly-like center. As long as these ligaments stay strong and unstretched, they can help to protect the discs. This is another reason to avoid extreme spinal movements.

When a disc herniates, it causes local inflammation, which hurts. In some cases, that's the worst thing that happens. In other cases, the herniated disc starts to put pressure on other structures near it. If those structures are the spinal cord or spinal nerves, then this is potentially a major problem.

That's why the most worrisome direction for a disc to herniate is backward, since the spinal cord is located behind the vertebral bodies. Because forward bends cause backward herniations (remember, the forward bend squishes the front of the disc, pushing the nucleus pulposus toward the back), it's most important to use caution with forward bending. As we'll explore in Chapter 7, the lumbar spine is particularly vulnerable to these types of herniations.

Imbibition

Hearing that extreme spinal movements can cause discs to herniate, you might feel tempted to minimize the movement of your spine, to protect your discs. However, that's not the best course of action. The reason is the way the discs receive their nutrients.

Once you're an adult, the discs don't have their own blood supply (like most other cartilage). They receive their nutrients and oxygen through a process known as imbibition – as in, they imbibe these things by soaking up the fluid that surrounds them. (This, too, is similar to other cartilage.)

For the discs to stay hydrated, they need to absorb this fluid. Movements of the spine squeeze the fluid into the various parts of the disc, keeping it healthy. That means that it's important to move the spine daily, in order to keep the discs from drying up. Tissue that becomes dry is more stiff and brittle, and more prone to being damaged. So even though there's a risk of herniating a disc when you bend the spine too deeply, keeping completely still is also a risky choice. Instead, frequent movement through your safe range of motion is optimal for the spine.

Facet Joints

The discs aren't the only point of contact between the vertebrae. Each vertebra contacts those above and below it at two small joints, called facet joints (fah-SET). Each bone has a flat surface, contacting a similar surface on the other bone. You can see these surfaces on the vertebrae in the illustration a few pages back; they look like small ovals of bone, between the spinous and transverse processes. The facet joints are synovial joints, with articular cartilage and joint capsules. Gliding movements occur between the two flat surfaces at these joints.

The orientation of the facet joints in each region of the spine determines the mobility of that region. The facet joints in the lumbar spine are oriented sagitally (i.e., vertical, and flat toward the middle of the body). This allows the lumbar spine to bend forward and backward quite easily, but rotation is very limited, because the spinal surfaces at the facet joints will run into each other as you try to twist. (Yoga teachers are used to telling you to "twist from your lower back," but the lower back actually twists very little in even the most mobile of backs.)

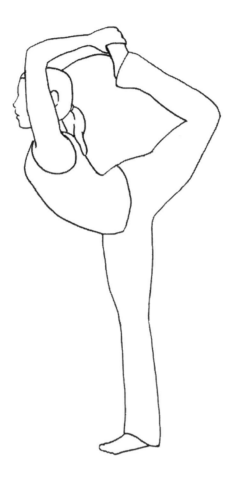

dancer's pose

The thoracic spine, on the other hand, has facet joints oriented obliquely. That allows it to side bend and rotate easily, but forward bending and backbending are more limited. In the central thoracic region, backbending is particularly limited, because the spinous processes point almost directly downwards, and are lying nearly on top of each other even when the spine is neutral. Backbending here is not possible. Look at people in a spinal extension like dancer's pose; even the most mobile backs have a region in the mid-back where the back is flat.

Understanding that the different regions of the spine are different will avoid a situation where you try to "work on" flexibility that will never come, potentially causing damage to the joints of that region. Trying to get your backbend deeper in your mid-back, or to twist deeper in your low back, will only lead to damage in these areas.

Posture

It's said that, as a river forms a canyon, "First the water shapes the land, and then the land shapes the water." Similarly, first your habits shape your body, and then your body shapes your habits. When you habitually hold a certain posture, it causes changes in your ligaments, tendons, and muscles; the changes are then self-reinforcing, because it's more comfortable to stand in your habitual posture than to choose a different shape. Once your body has become accustomed to a certain posture, changing it takes effort. It's worth it, though, to keep your back and neck feeling great.

To check your posture, stand with your back against a wall. Once your back is on the wall, notice the back of your head. If your cervical curve is healthy, the back of your head should be touching the wall. This will place your ears directly over your shoulders.

Many people find that their heads are forward, not touching the wall. This is colloquially referred to as "turtle neck" by many yoga teachers and physical therapists. It's a combination of a forward bend in your lower cervical spine (which thrusts the head forward), and a backbend in your upper cervical spine (which allows you to look forward instead of at the floor). If you have neck pain, chances are very good that this is your neck's normal position. I find that if I spend a lot of time at the computer for a few days, I start to get turtle neck.

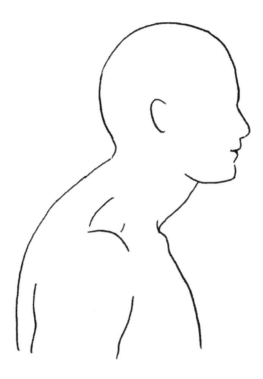

turtle neck

Trying to backbend a neck that's already in the turtle neck position will almost never feel good. People will describe feeling crowding in the neck as they try to bend it backward. If you slide your head back first, bringing your ears over your shoulders and aligning your cervical spine, and *then* try to backbend your neck, you may find that you have a lot more room in your neck. (Still, use caution with backbends of the neck, as we'll discuss in the next chapter.)

Next, try to slide your hand behind your low back. Ideally, you want your fingers to slide in, but to get stuck at the knuckles. This is a rough approximation of a healthy lumbar curve.

If you find that your fingers can't slide behind your low back, then you have an overly rounded low back, and should work on increasing your lumbar curve to a healthy state. This is common in those who spend a lot of time in chairs that don't have lumbar support. Now that companies are more aware of ergonomics, most chairs do have lumbar support, so work may be a less common source of low back rounding. At the same time, anyone who sits on a couch in the evenings is at risk for this problem.

Some people find that they can slide their whole hand, and maybe even their whole arm, behind their low back. This indicates a lumbar curve that's hyperextended, meaning that your low back is arched too far forward. This is particularly common in women who have been pregnant (even years before), although it can happen in anyone. The low back hyperextension happens because the core muscles of the abdomen aren't strong, and so the weight of the abdomen and its organs falls forward instead of being supported by the abdominal wall. This weight pulls forward on the spine, causing it to arch. Over time, with an overly arched low back, the discs and joints of the lumbar spine, as well as the tendons, ligaments, and muscles of the area, will end up strained and tender.

If your low back is already overly arched forward, then working on backbends in this area will only make your problem worse. It might be tempting to do a super-deep wheel pose, but it will just add more damage to your already-tender low back. If you have a hyperextended low back, you're better off avoiding any deep backbending of this area, instead keeping your tailbone tucked as you do backbends to make them less deep.

While you're at the wall for your posture check, why not take advantage of that wall? Many of my students LOVE using a tennis ball as a little self-massager. With your back still on the wall, put your tennis ball behind your low back, your glutes, your upper back, or between your shoulder blade and your spine. Lean back onto it and gently move around to massage the area, tennis ball rolling along any tight or sore areas.

The only place to avoid is the mid-back, right near the bottom of your ribs; this is where your kidneys are located, and pressing into them too much is not good for them. Otherwise, massage wherever you feel like you need to. Putting the tennis ball directly on bone won't feel good, for the most part (although the sacrum is generally an exception), so stay mainly on the muscles. This exercise is frequently requested in my classes!

Symmetry

Almost no one stands completely symmetrically at all times. We usually lean our weight more on one leg than on the other. When we sit, we often cross one leg over the other, and it's usually the same leg on top every time. When we sleep, we may lie on one side preferentially (especially when a partner is sharing the bed).

During yoga class, standing symmetrically is generally emphasized. However, if you spend the other 23 hours of your day in an asymmetrical posture, then even going to yoga class every day will probably not keep your spine optimally healthy.

When you're in mountain pose (tadasana), work on standing completely symmetrically, with your spine tall and normal curves present but not exaggerated. Do your best to memorize this shape. Anytime you remember throughout your day, bring yourself back to the same feeling in your spine (whether you're standing or sitting).

Slowly, over time, you'll find that your new habits reshape your body. As water is diverted, it carves new channels. Soon, good alignment of your spine will become a habit. While it may seem like just another thing you have to pay attention to, the benefits of an aligned spine are worth the effort. Some studies have even indicated improvements in mood when people are in a well-aligned posture, as compared to when they're hunching or slouching.

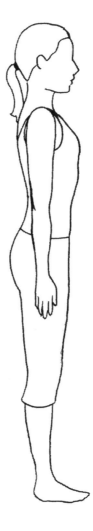

tadasana

Sleeping

You spend about eight hours in bed every night. (Right? If not, then you should. Sleep is excellent for your health!) The position in which you sleep will have a significant impact on the health of your spine. During sleep, your muscle tone is very low, so your joints can't be protected by muscular effort; that means you need to position your body carefully to prevent yourself from ending up with back pain.

Many people choose to sleep while lying on their sides, and many of those prefer one side over the other, especially if they have a spouse or partner who shares their bed. (I call this the "spooning effect.") When you and your partner each choose a side of the bed to be "your" side, you'll tend to develop an asymmetry in which side you sleep on. For some couples, periodically switching who sleeps on which side can help to relieve this problem.

In order to keep your back healthy, you want to prevent your spine from curving to one side or the other during sleep. One aspect of this is having a pillow that aligns your neck properly; you may need to search around until you find one that's the right height. On your side, your neck should be parallel to the ground; on your back, your normal cervical curve should be maintained.

You also want to support the alignment of your thoracic and lumbar spine. Some mattresses are able to absorb your weight and hold your spine in good alignment while you sleep on your side. If yours doesn't, then it might help to place a small pillow (like a couch pillow, or even a folded towel) under your side waist, so there's no sagging of your spine down into the bed.

It's also important to keep the knees and hips aligned, to prevent damage to the SI joints. That means putting a pillow between the knees *and* ankles, so the legs are parallel and the low back is happy. We'll discuss this more in Chapter 7.

How to Protect Your Back

- Keep your forward, back, and side bends out of the extreme range, never pushing into any area that's tender, to protect your intervertebral discs.

- Don't push your twists and forward bends (such as plow pose) too deep, to protect the ligaments of your spine.
- Be aware that different regions of the spine move differently. Don't try to achieve deep twists in the low back or backbends in the mid back, to protect the facet joints between the vertebrae.
- Work toward aligning your posture, minimizing any asymmetry between left and right, and protecting the natural curves of your spine, to protect all of the tissues of your back. Bring awareness to your posture throughout the day and as you go to sleep.

We've explored the spine in general. In the next two chapters, we'll look at specific regions of the spine that require extra consideration. Let's explore the neck, an area containing many important structures. A rare but devastating injury can occur if you don't know how to protect your neck during yoga practice.

CHAPTER 6:
THE NECK

If your neck sometimes feels stiff or sore by the end of the day, you're not alone. Unfortunately, the neck is a common source of discomfort in modern society. As discussed in Chapter 5, "turtle neck" is a major contributor to this situation. Hunching in the mid-back contributes to this turtle neck position, and looking down at electronic devices worsens the neck's situation. Our modern environment is definitely not designed to support neck health.

Because of all of these forces, many yoga practitioners mention reducing neck stiffness as a goal for their yoga practice. With more and more people spending their work days at computers, I'd expect this goal to become even more common. Yoga certainly has the potential to help keep your neck healthy in a variety of ways.

However, the neck contains several delicate structures, and it's important to know how to protect them as you practice, or you risk increasing neck pain – or worse. Let's begin our exploration of the neck with a look at the cervical spine.

The Cervical Spine

As mentioned in the previous chapter, there are 7 vertebrae in the neck, known as C1 through C7. These cervical vertebrae have small, delicate bodies, as they don't have to support much body weight. The last cervical vertebra, C7, has a longer spinous process than the ones above it; this is called vertebra prominens (think "prominent"). If you run your finger lightly along the back of your neck, it's easy to distinguish this landmark. You can feel how the forward curve of your neck turns into the backward curve of your mid-back below C7.

The top two vertebrae are different from the others. C1, also known as the atlas, has no vertebral body. The skull rests in C1 like a cup in a saucer. The only movement possible here is the "yes" movement (nodding the head), with the skull tipping back and forth on C1.

C2 essentially has a double vertebral body, having acquired its extra one from C1 during embryonic life. It sticks up from the main C2 vertebral body like a tooth, and fits into a small ring on C1. (There's no disc between these two vertebrae as a result of this vertebral body migration.) C1 rotates on C2 to create the "no" movement (shaking the head). If you make very small "yes" and "no" movements and tune into subtle sensations, you might be able to feel them occurring in slightly different places in your neck. Larger movements start to involve the whole neck, making it harder to feel that small and subtle difference.

The facet joints of the cervical spine allow for a wide range of movements, and the cervical region is the most mobile part of the spine. When the spine is in a combination of a backbend and a side bend, the facet joints are slightly pulled apart (this is known as "distraction"), destabilizing the cervical spine. This is one reason that head circles, where the head is rolled all the way around on the neck, are not recommended. However, as we're about to explore, there's an even more important reason to avoid head circles.

The Vertebral Arteries

The transverse processes of the cervical vertebrae are distinct from those in the rest of the spine. Within each transverse process is a small hole. Stacking these together creates a channel that runs through each side of the cervical spine. In these channels are the two vertebral arteries, which are important in supplying blood to the brain.

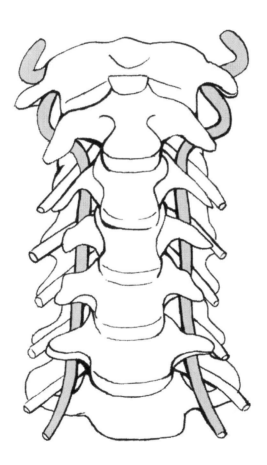

vertebral arteries (highlighted in gray) with the cervical spine; the white structures are the spinal nerves

When the neck is in a position of backbending plus rotation, or backbending plus side bending, these arteries are at risk. This position can pinch the vertebral arteries. In the moment, this can slow or even stop blood flow through the artery. Some people may feel dizzy when that happens, because of reduced blood flow to the brain.

For many people, however, the reduction of blood flow actually won't cause any noticeable symptoms. That's because the blood flow to the brain is designed with redundancies, since it's so crucial to keep the brain supplied with blood to maintain consciousness. The two vertebral arteries and the two carotid arteries (the large arteries you can feel in the front of the neck) meet in a circle at the base of the brain, where they share their blood. From this circle, the arteries that carry blood to the brain arise.

Because of the sharing of blood in this circle, pinching off one vertebral artery doesn't have a huge impact on the blood flow to the brain; blood simply flows through the other arteries, and consciousness is maintained.

However, this ability to maintain blood flow doesn't mean that pinching the vertebral arteries is okay. When an artery is pinched, its wall is often damaged. Where there's a damaged artery wall, a blood clot will form, both because exposed arterial wall cells begin the clotting process and because the blood flow near the injury is usually altered in such a way that some of the blood stagnates. In some cases, part of the lining of the artery peels away from the arterial wall, forming a little stagnant pocket of blood. Stagnant blood often clots.

If a clot is formed on the vertebral artery wall near where it was pinched, a race against time begins. The body may dissolve the clot before anything bad happens, and repair the damage to the artery. But if part of the clot breaks off and is carried by the flowing blood up into the brain, it results in a stroke. The clot gets stuck in a smaller artery and blocks off the flow of blood there, depriving a part of the brain of oxygen and nutrients and potentially damaging or killing the brain cells there.

Again, because the reduction in blood flow through the vertebral artery doesn't necessarily cause any obvious effects, you may not know in the moment if your artery is being pinched. When the damage becomes obvious is minutes or hours later, when the stroke happens.

While backbending plus rotation (or backbending plus side bending) is the most dangerous position the neck can be in, deep forward bending plus rotation (or deep forward bending plus side bending) is also a precarious position for the vertebral arteries. Even a very deep backbend of the neck without rotation or side bending can lead to pinching the vertebral arteries. (This last has been termed "beauty parlor stroke syndrome," because some of the sinks at which salons wash clients' hair cause very deep backbends of the neck.)

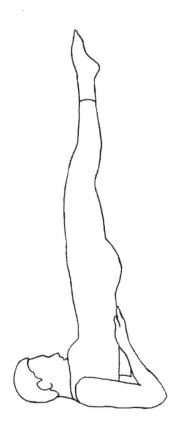

shoulderstand

Shoulderstand and plow are very deep flexions of the neck, with extra force from the body weight being loaded onto the neck. Looking sideways in these poses – as new students are very likely to do, because they want to see if they're doing the pose right – is potentially dangerous for the vertebral arteries. If you're teaching a yoga class, be sure that you warn students about this issue. You can tell them that if they want to look around the room, they should come out of the pose first, look, and then go back in, rather than putting their necks at risk by looking around from within the pose.

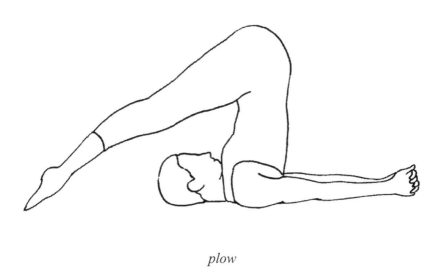

plow

Dropping the head back in camel is potentially a risky move as well. With gravity pulling the head backward, the potential for excessively deep neck extension is clear. The older the student, the more careful he or she should be about the neck, because arteries tend to stiffen with age, making them more vulnerable to damage. Camel is risky on the low back, too (because of the pull of gravity), so you could avoid this pose and replace it with other backbends (as I do). If you choose to do camel, consider protecting the neck by not dropping the head all the way back. If the person in this illustration were a yoga student in my class, I'd have some concern about both her low back and her neck, as they're both in deep extension.

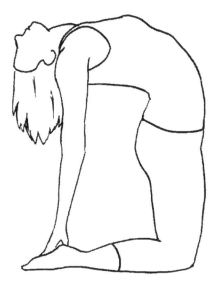

camel pose

Sometimes, the neck risk is less obvious. For example, consider a seated twist. Recall from Chapter 5 that many people have excessive thoracic flexion (hunching forward in the mid-back and shoulders), and resultant cervical extension (backbending of the neck, aka "turtle neck"). If a twist is initiated from this spinal alignment, then the neck will be put into a risky position of backbend plus twist. This is why it's important to cue students to align their spines vertically before twisting.

I don't want to cause unnecessary alarm. Even when placed in a risky position, a stroke resulting from vertebral artery compression is a rare event, and only a few documented cases have ever occurred due to yoga practice. However, some of these have unfortunately occurred in young, healthy people who never expected an event like that. We should not accept any cases of vertebral artery compression in yoga, when an understanding of how to protect the neck could prevent them.

Blood Pressure

The vertebral arteries in the sides of the cervical spine are only two of the four arteries supplying the brain with blood. The other two are the carotid arteries, which are larger than the vertebral arteries. You can feel the pulse of these arteries by laying your fingers gently on your neck; on the front of the neck, just inside of the sternocleidomastoid muscle that runs diagonally down to your collarbone, is the easiest place to find the carotid pulse.

Now, let's consider the brain. There's a rigid boundary (the skull) that defines the space within which the brain rests. Since this space can't be expanded, its volume is fixed. In this fixed volume, there are three main things.

1. Cerebrospinal fluid. This is a fluid, and therefore not compressible.
2. Blood. Again, a fluid, not compressible.
3. Brain tissue. When this is compressed, there are consequences!

In general, the body does a great job of maintaining blood flow to the brain within strict parameters. Too little, and consciousness can't be maintained; too much, and there will be brain damage from the increased pressure. When you put your head below your heart, gravity acts to pull extra blood into your brain. The arteries to the brain constrict (close down slightly) to resist this pull, and the overall blood flow to the brain doesn't increase. (So there is no "extra blood/oxygen flowing to your brain" when you're upside down, despite the prevalence of this statement in yoga classes. Though the changed perspective can be pretty inspiring.)

The blood flow to your face doesn't require strict control like this. Because of that, turning upside down can result in increased blood flow to the face, as every yoga practitioner who's ever disliked a picture of themselves in an inversion can attest. The brain, however, is protected.

However, this system has a limit. When the blood pressure exceeds this limit, the arteries become unable to hold back the extra blood. The pressure inside the skull cavity starts to rise, and brain damage can occur.

(We're about to discuss high blood pressure, so I just want to reiterate: this book is not intended to provide you with medical advice. If you have high blood pressure or any other medical condition, please discuss your yoga practice with your own doctor. It may help, however, to understand the issues involved.)

Consider someone who already has high blood pressure when they're upright. In most cases, their blood pressure is elevated, but is still within the limits of the system; the blood flow to the brain is still relatively well-controlled. (If it isn't, because the blood pressure is above the limit even while upright, that should be treated immediately.) When this person with elevated blood pressure inverts (puts the head below the heart), and gravity adds extra pressure to that already-high blood pressure, then the limits of the system may be exceeded. The arteries won't be able to hold back that extra blood, because the total pressure is too high for the arteries to resist. The pressure inside the skull will rise, and brain damage can result.

That's why people who have high blood pressure should completely avoid inversions. That doesn't just mean headstand and handstand; it means any pose where the head is below the heart, including such beginner-friendly poses as downward dog and standing forward fold. Any of these have the potential to raise blood pressure past a critical point in people who already have high blood pressure.

Keep in mind that by "people who have high blood pressure," I mean "people whose blood pressure is high right now." Many people who say that they "have high blood pressure" mean that they take medication to keep their blood pressure in the normal range. If you're on these medications, and your blood pressure is normal, then inverting is likely to be safe for you. If you have significant variations in your blood pressure, it's a good idea to take your blood pressure before you go to yoga class (or at least once every morning), so that you can protect your brain by avoiding inversions if it happens to be high that day. (Many other things besides inversions can also raise blood pressure, and are dangerous too; discussing them all is beyond the scope of this book.)

When someone is diagnosed with high blood pressure, he or she may want to try lifestyle modifications before starting on a medication. This is a great choice, and it's very likely to work – in the long run. Yoga as part of an exercise and stress-reduction plan has been shown in studies to be effective in lowering blood pressure. But when a newly-diagnosed person walks into their first yoga class, it's very important for that person to avoid inversions throughout class.

That can mean simple modifications, like placing the hands on a block to keep the spine parallel to the ground in a forward fold rather than allowing the full fold with the head down.

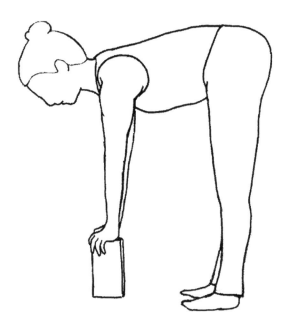

modified forward fold

Sometimes it takes more creativity; replacing a pose like downward dog in a flow can be a challenge, and sometimes the modified transitions may feel a little awkward. You could try replacing downward dog with plank pose.

The pressure in the eyes can go up when you invert, so those with glaucoma are also advised to avoid inversions. There are also a few other conditions that would make inversions unsafe for you. If you have high blood pressure or any other medical condition, please talk with your doctor about your yoga practice, to get personalized medical advice for your situation.

Body Weight on the Head

Few issues in yoga are more controversial than the issue of headstand. Some practitioners believe it's unsafe, while others fiercely defend their right and their ability to do headstands safely. Let's look at the issues involved, so you can make your own decision.

The cervical vertebrae are the smallest in the body. They normally bear only the weight of the head, which is a few pounds. When you compare the cervical vertebrae with the lumbar vertebrae, it's clear that the lumbar vertebrae are much larger and thicker, which allows them to bear more weight safely. The cervical vertebrae are not designed to do this.

I've heard it said that people in certain countries carry a significant amount of weight on top of their heads regularly, proving that the neck can handle more than just the weight of the head. Keep in mind that the people in these societies have carried weight on their heads from a young age, so their bones have developed the shape and density to handle doing so. Those of us in Western societies who begin to work toward headstand are loading most of our body weight onto our delicate cervical vertebrae with virtually no ramp-up.

Also, while some studies of these populations have shown no increase in neck problems, other studies have shown that societies where people routinely carry things on their heads have a significantly increased rate of neck problems. Just because people do something doesn't mean that it's good for them. In many cases, they simply have no choice.

If you choose to practice headstand, it's ideal to keep as much of the weight in your arms as possible. Even in those societies that carry things on their heads, they carry up to 70% of their body weight – not all of it. With your vertebrae not adapted over your lifetime to handle very heavy loads, you should be aiming for much less than 70%. Press with your hands or arms, using the strength of those muscles to hold most of your weight.

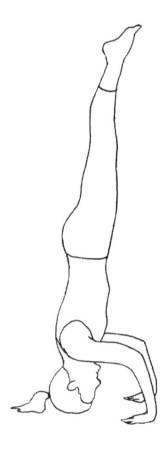

tripod headstand

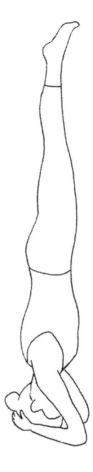

bound headstand

That may cause your body not to be exactly perpendicular to the ground, but the aesthetics of the pose are far less important than the effect on your neck. If your spine is completely vertical, then most of your body weight will end up in your neck, which isn't ideal. This is especially true in tripod headstand; there's no way to shift your weight into your arms while keeping your spine vertical in this pose. In bound headstand, it's possible to keep the spine closer to vertical while bearing the weight in the arms, by hovering the head slightly above the ground. Yoga teachers tend to chastise their students for aligning their headstands at a slight angle rather than completely vertically, but that instruction is based in aesthetics rather than safety.

Also, use a wall while you're learning headstand. If you're wobbly, serious neck injuries can occur when your neck bends quickly while it's loaded with weight. The arteries, tendons, or ligaments may be damaged, a disc may rupture, and it's even possible to fracture the spine if you fall out of a headstand. It's unsafe to practice headstand away from a wall until you're completely stable every time.

I feel that headstand should virtually never be taught in a group class. When a yoga teacher says something like, "You can take a headstand if it's in your practice," the implication is that you should be in a headstand if you're good at yoga, and many yoga students will attempt to do so even though they aren't really prepared. Even if they're warned about this danger, people will still be tempted to show off, or to "win yoga class" by doing the most advanced poses. If you're a student and a teacher says this, be mindful of this desire if it arises (let's face it, we're socialized to push ourselves hard and compete), and then resist it for your own protection.

I believe that this pose should only be taught in a workshop format, or in an advanced class in which the teacher knows every student and feels confident that everyone is safe in the pose. If you want to teach it in a group class, I recommend that you stop the flow of class, show the alignment, and work with each student as necessary to ensure that they're doing the pose safely. To flow through it with simply an "if it's in your practice" type of instruction is to invite students to take dangerous risks. (Some of them will take those risks, even if you tell them not to.)

You may also choose to avoid this pose, as a teacher or as a practitioner, because the biomechanics of the pose put unnatural loads on the delicate cervical spine and you don't want to risk neck problems. You definitely don't have to practice headstand in order to be a yogi. Many advanced practitioners avoid this pose, considering its benefits not to be worth the risks. This is a completely rational choice; it's not "living from fear," but rather mindfully choosing from a place of knowledge. Please feel empowered to make this choice, if it's the right path for you. If you receive significant benefits from headstand and you want to do the pose, please ensure that you do so as safely as possible.

How To Protect Your Neck

- Restrict the depth of backbends and forward bends of the neck, to avoid overly stretching the neck's supporting ligaments as well as to protect the vertebral arteries.
- Avoid combining a backbend with a side bend or rotation of the neck, as this could damage the vertebral arteries and lead to a stroke. A deep forward bend plus side bend or rotation can cause the same problem.
- If you have high blood pressure, avoid any pose where your head is below your heart, until your blood pressure is brought under control. If you have any medical condition (including high blood pressure), please talk with your doctor about your yoga practice to ensure that you stay safe.
- If you choose to practice headstand, use the strength of the arms to minimize the amount of weight in your head, and only enter the pose if you feel completely stable.

The neck is one of the common problem areas of the spine. The other area that can require special protection is the low back. With a huge proportion of American adults reporting that they experience low back pain, it pays to learn more about how you can protect this region of your spine. In the next chapter, we'll explore it.

CHAPTER 7:
THE LOW BACK

It seems that almost everyone has low back issues. When I ask my yoga students what's bothering them on a given day, it's guaranteed that a few people will say that their lower back is stiff, sore, or both.

Official estimates indicate that up to 80% of American adults will experience significant low back pain at some point in their lives. For many, it's bad enough to make them stay home from work or school.

Low back pain is a common reason for people to begin a yoga practice. Of course, this book is not intended to provide treatment for any pain that you have; discuss it with your doctor or physical therapist to get individualized recommendations. But I can offer you tips for keeping your low back healthy as you practice.

The Lumbar Spine

The vertebrae in the lumbar spine are the largest ones, because they have to bear the body weight. That amount of force being applied to this region daily is one reason that the lumbar spine is particularly vulnerable to injury. Even though the vertebral bodies are thick and strong, the discs and ligaments are subjected to a lot of strain from the body weight.

Additionally, the lumbar spine is relatively unsupported. Recall from Chapter 5 that the longitudinal ligaments run vertically along the front and back of the bodies of the vertebrae, helping to hold them in alignment and also to protect the discs from herniation. Toward the bottom of the spinal column, these ligaments become much thinner. That means there's less support for the vertebrae and the discs in this region, despite the extra force they need to bear.

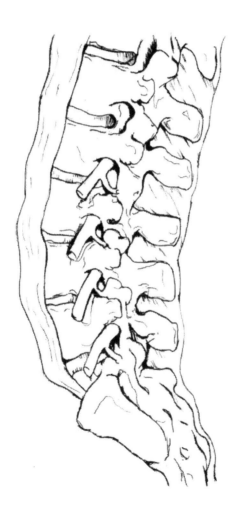

the lumbar spine

Also, at the bottom of the spine, between L5 and the sacrum, there's a sharp shift in the angle of curvature. Gravity is attempting to pull the lumbar spine forward and off the sacrum, in exactly the part of the spine that's least supported by connective tissue. That makes this part of the back vulnerable to damage.

Herniation of the discs of the lumbar spine is most common when the lumbar spine is in flexion (a forward bend), particularly when it's loaded with weight. This is why people are told to lift heavy objects using their legs, rather than bending over and lifting from their back; keeping the low back in slight extension (a small backbend) helps to protect it.

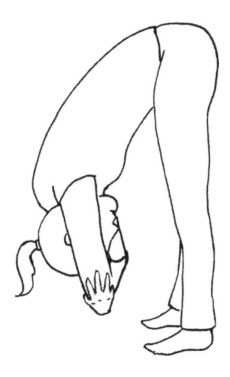

standing forward bend

Actually, a pose like standing forward bend includes lumbar flexion loaded with weight – the weight of the upper body. It would be rare for a yoga practitioner to herniate a lumbar disc during the practice of a pose like this; it usually takes more weight, such as a heavy box, to cause a herniation. Still, forcing the lumbar spine into extreme flexion is not a good idea; it will tend to put a lot of pressure on the discs, potentially wearing them down over time and making them more likely to have problems later.

In poses like this one, yoga students will sometimes force extreme lumbar flexion as they try their best to touch their toes (or palm the floor, depending on where they are in their yoga journey). That's why I like the variation where the practitioner holds opposite elbows, as in the illustration; it removes the temptation to force oneself to touch the toes.

The Thoracolumbar Fascia

In the lower back, there's a diamond-shaped region where the tendons of many muscles come together to form a thick layer of connective tissue. This type of structure is called an aponeurosis; structurally, it's a big flat tendon. In the low back, this aponeurosis is called the thoracolumbar fascia.

You can see this structure in the illustration on the next page; it's the big white area in the lower back. The muscles below it are the gluteus maximus (the big muscles of the buttocks). To each side is latissimus dorsi, and above it are the trapezius muscles, which we'll discuss in Chapter 8. Several other muscles also attach to the thoracolumbar fascia.

The thoracolumbar fascia is stretched by forward bending. When people perform excessively deep forward bends (such as when they first begin a yoga practice and can't touch their toes), they can strain the thoracolumbar fascia, which will be felt as a general ache in the lower back. In addition to the risk to the discs, this is another reason to use caution in forward bends, staying away from any action that forces this movement to be very deep.

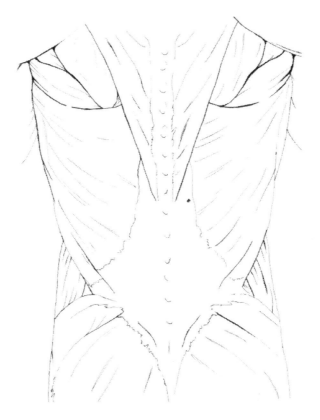

thoracolumbar fascia

Problems in this region aren't restricted to those who are new to yoga. Any yoga practitioner could strain this area by forcing themselves into a deep forward bend. This is common in practitioners who take a break from their yoga practice, and find that they've lost some flexibility; they may "work" to get their range of motion back to its previous level, and can strain the thoracolumbar fascia in the process. Anytime someone decides to "work on" a pose that requires hip flexion, they may end up straining the low back, as rounding of the lumbar spine is used to make up for a lack of hip flexibility.

If there's excessive pressure in the low back in a forward bend, there are two options for relieving it. You could come up out of the pose until the low back feels better. You could also bend the knees, which will release the tension on the hamstrings and allow the pelvis to tip forward; this will also decrease the amount of flexion in the low back. However you accomplish it, you should ensure that the amount of flexion in your lumbar spine is not excessive, or many structures may be at risk.

Sympathetic Curves

Try a little exercise: lie on your back, with your knees bent. Notice your low back; there should be a little space behind it (your lumbar curve). Press your low back toward the floor, eliminating that space.

Now, notice your neck. Did the back of your neck also come toward the floor?

The cervical and lumbar curves are known as sympathetic curves. That means that they tend to move together. When one flexes (does a forward bend), the other will tend to flex along with it; the same with extension (backbending). This is just a tendency, and can be unlearned as you acquire more precise body control. However, it can be a useful tendency.

When you're coming into a forward bend, you should be aiming to prevent your lumbar spine from going into the deepest possible flexion, as this could strain the structures of the low back. You want to restrict the flexion of your lumbar spine a bit. The sympathetic nature of the cervical and lumbar curves can help you do that.

For instance, as you go into a seated forward bend, you could look forward slightly, toward your feet. This is an extension of the cervical spine, which will tend to create a corresponding extension of the lumbar spine. Keeping the neck in that backbend as you enter the pose will tend to keep the lumbar spine slightly away from its very deepest flexion. Once you reach a safe edge for the stretch, you can drop the tension in your neck – as long as you don't then deepen the stretch in the low back, which would undo the benefits of this technique. Find your edge, then stay there as you relax the neck.

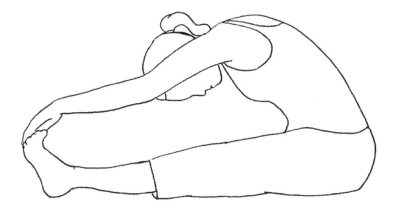

seated forward fold

It's not a guarantee, but using your sympathetic curves in ways like this could help protect you from overdoing it in the low back. If you're a teacher, you can also cue this in your classes to help your students stay protected, as many students have a strong tendency to push themselves in forward bends during yoga class.

The Sacrum

There are five vertebrae in the sacral region of the spine. During embryology, these five fuse together into one bone, called the sacrum. This bone is shaped like a flat triangle with several holes in it; the holes occur in the places where two vertebrae have fused together, and spinal nerves pass through these holes (much like they pass through the foramina between each pair of vertebrae in other spinal regions). The triangle is wider at the top, and it tapers to become smaller toward the tailbone. Additionally, the sacrum is curved toward the back of the body (in the same direction as the thoracic spine).

There are two or three very tiny vertebral remnants below the sacrum, which fuse together to make the tailbone, or coccyx (COCK-six). While it's tempting to think of the tailbone as "vestigial," meaning that it's just a remnant of a tail with no purpose, the tailbone is actually very important in supporting the muscles of the pelvic floor. The tailbone curves in the same direction as the sacrum, with its end pointing inward.

The Pelvis

While it may seem as though it's one bone, the pelvis is actually made up of two separate bones, one on each side. These bones are called the innominate bones, which means "the bones with no name." Apparently their complicated shape made it too hard for those early anatomists to choose a name for them. (At least they didn't decide to just give them the same name as some other completely different structure.)

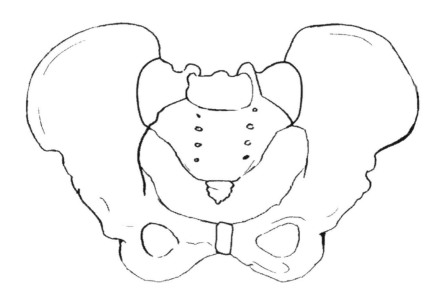

the pelvis, sacrum, and coccyx

Each innominate bone is actually formed from the fusion of three bones, called the ilium, the ischium, and the pubis. Before puberty, these are separate bones; at puberty, they fuse together to make one innominate bone. The names for various structures in the pelvis are related to which bone formed that structure. For instance, the "sitting bones" are officially called the ischial tuberosities, because they're initially part of the ischium.

The two innominate bones join in the front at the pubic symphysis. This is a cartilaginous joint, containing a disc of fibrocartilage very similar in structure to the intervertebral discs (the ones between the vertebrae). Also like the intervertebral discs, the disc at the pubic symphysis is attached on both sides to the bone. That gives this joint a limited ability to move. The only movements that can occur there are those that squish the disc; the two bones can move slightly closer together or farther away, and they can also twist slightly relative to each other.

There is another joint made by each of the innominate bones. That's the joint made at the back of the pelvis with the sacrum, the triangular bone of the lower back. This is the SI joint.

The SI Joints

The sacrum rests within the pelvis, between the two pelvic bones. It's a triangle resting in a triangular-shaped space. When you're upright, gravity helps to hold the sacrum in place by pulling it down into that space, helping keep this part of the low back stable.

The sacrum forms a synovial joint with each innominate bone. These joints are called the SI joints (SI is for sacroinnominate, although they're sometimes called the sacroiliac joints, because they're initially part of the ilium; SI works for either version). Each SI joint is about the size of your thumb.

The SI joints are stabilized by plenty of connective tissue. Many strong ligaments attach to the sacrum and the pelvis, both in the front and in the back.   In this joint, stability is the most important feature. However, movements of the SI joints are possible.

The movements that can happen here are called nutation and counternutation. They essentially involve rotating the sacrum around the axis created by the two joints. When the top of the sacrum tips forward and the bottom tips backward, that's nutation; when the opposite occurs, it's counternutation. Basically, counternutation is tucking the tailbone, while nutation is untucking the tailbone.

These movements are so small that there was debate for some time about whether any movement at the SI joints was actually possible. It turns out that it is, but it's normally small and subtle. Larger movements of the SI joints can damage them. Women commonly notice discomfort in their SI joints during pregnancy, when hormones make connective tissue looser, allowing the SI joints to move more than they normally would.

If you feel discomfort in one of your SI joints, it's usually a one-sided sensation occurring in your lower back, around the side of your sacrum, but deeper. This contrasts with discomfort in the thoracolumbar fascia, which affects the low back more generally, or discomfort in the lumbar spine, which will be in the middle of the back. It's helpful to know what to feel for, so that you can address the problem and prevent damage to the joint.

By moving the two halves of the pelvis, the rotation of the hips also affects the SI joint, so the placement of your hips is crucial to your low back health. We'll discuss this more in Chapter 11.

Pelvic Rotation

Imagine the pelvis as a bowl. When the bowl tips forward, that's called anteversion; the bowl would be spilling toward the front of your body, and your tailbone would be moving back. When the bowl tips backward, that's called retroversion; imagine the bowl spilling behind you, and your pubic bone moving up toward your navel. When the pelvis is neutral, the points on the fronts of your hip crests (known as your ASIS bones) and your pubic symphysis will be in the same vertical plane.

The rotation of the pelvis, the movements of the sacrum, and the position of the lumbar spine are all linked together. This linkage is known as lumbosacral rhythm. It's created by the ways that these structures are put together, meaning that you can't learn not to do it (unlike the sympathetic spinal curve movements of the cervical and lumbar spine). Knowledge of lumbosacral rhythm allows you to protect your lower back during yoga and the rest of your activities.

These movements go together: pelvic anteversion (the pelvis tipping forward), sacral nutation (the tailbone moving backward as the top of the sacrum moves forward), and lumbar extension (backbending in the lower back).

That means that these movements also go together: pelvic retroversion (the pelvis tipping backward), sacral counternutation (the tailbone tucking as the top of the sacrum moves backward), and lumbar flexion (rounding of the low back).

If your lumbar spine is experiencing too much extension or flexion, you can address it using lumbosacral rhythm. Let's look at an example.

Lumbar Hyperextension

Many people chronically have too much extension in the low back. This can result from weak abs; because the abdominal muscles pull the pelvis into retroversion (by pulling upwards on the pubic symphysis), they also cause lumbar flexion (rounding of the lower back). When they're weak, then the lumbar spine tends to fall into hyperextension.

Women commonly develop lumbar hyperextension during pregnancy, because of the weight of the baby and the overstretching of the abs. Often, this condition persists even after pregnancy, often for years, with the lumbar hyperextension causing back pain. The abdominal muscles become separated from each other, and putting them back together is difficult. Pushing into this with deep backbends of the lower back will make things worse.

If you already have a hyperextended lumbar spine, then adding backbends of your low back will only make the problem worse. Even if your lumbar spine doesn't have this problem, backbending very deeply can injure the discs, ligaments, or other tissues of the spine. Pushing into backbends in this region is likely to lead to injury.

Let's consider a spinal extension pose. When you go into camel pose, you extend the whole spine. The tendency of gravity is to pull the spine into deeper extension, as the weight of your upper body tilts backward. This pose can be dangerous, because unless you use muscular strength to oppose this gravitational pull, it's very easy to hyperextend, injuring the low back.

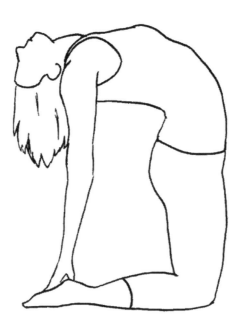

camel pose

To protect the low back, you can use lumbosacral rhythm. Before you begin backbending into camel pose, tuck your tailbone slightly. This tips the pelvis backward and also flexes (rounds) the lumbar spine. Keep the tailbone tucked as you allow yourself to bend backward into the pose. This pull of the lumbar spine slightly toward flexion prevents it from going into an extension that's too deep.

This can be useful in any backbends. If you want to do the deepest possible backbend (for instance, for a photo shoot), then you'll need to untuck your tailbone and tip your pelvis forward, to allow for the deepest possible backbend in your lower back. Keeping your tailbone tucked as you go into a backbend will prevent full extension of your lumbar spine, so your backbend won't be as deep. However, if you want to protect your lower back from becoming hyperextended, then a slight tuck of your tailbone as you come into the pose will help to prevent your lower back from becoming too extended.

In other words, tuck your tailbone a little when you backbend, because this will make it harder to backbend.

The Psoas

The psoas (SO-az) is, in my teaching experience, the biggest muscle most people have never heard of.

It's a muscle of the core, but because of its location, it's not an obvious one. It attaches to the bodies of the lumbar vertebrae (which, of course, are hidden inside the body). The psoas then passes down and forward, crosses the bowl of the pelvis, and attaches inside of the femur (the thighbone). In the illustration of the psoas below, you're looking at the back of the body from the inside. The front of the body and all of the abdominal organs are gone, so you can see the psoas. The structure above the psoas is the diaphragm; toward the middle of the body is the spine (the vertebral bodies, covered in the anterior longitudinal ligament).

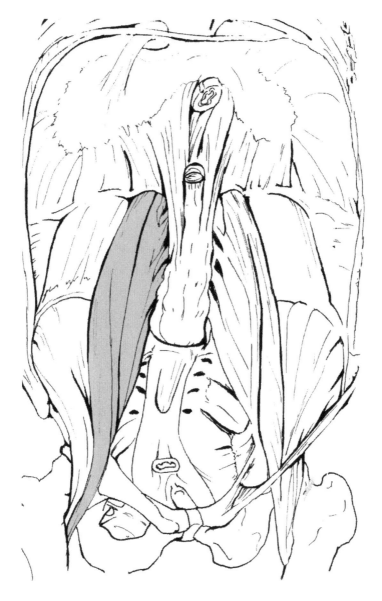

psoas (highlighted in gray)

The main function of the psoas is to flex the hip (i.e., bring the thigh toward the torso). That means that the psoas is shortened when the hip is flexed, such as when you're sitting. Most of us spend an awful lot of time sitting – that's how our built environment is designed. When you put a muscle into a shortened position for a long time, it has a tendency to become tight; in people who sit a lot, a tight psoas is common.

If you have a tight psoas, and then you stand up (extending your hips and stretching your psoas), your psoas will pull on the inside of your lower back. It will create tension in your lumbar spine, pulling it into extension and the pelvis into anteversion. This may lead to low back discomfort.

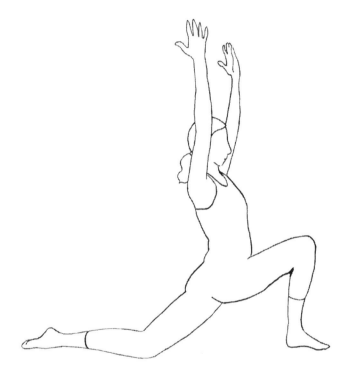

low lunge, sagging weight forward

For many people, the low back feels better when they stretch the hips. Hip extension will lengthen the psoas (because the psoas is a hip flexor). Because it pulls the pelvis into anteversion when it contracts, the psoas is also stretched by putting the pelvis into retroversion (i.e., tucking the tailbone).

Low lunge is a psoas stretch, and can be very helpful for keeping the low back happy. There are two ways to do low lunge. The first one (shown on the previous page) is the way people do it in photo shoots, because it looks deeper – you let your weight sag forward to create extension in the back hip. However, you can see that there's a lot of lumbar extension in this version. For those who already have back pain due to psoas-induced lumbar hyperextension, this is not going to be a very productive way to fix the problem.

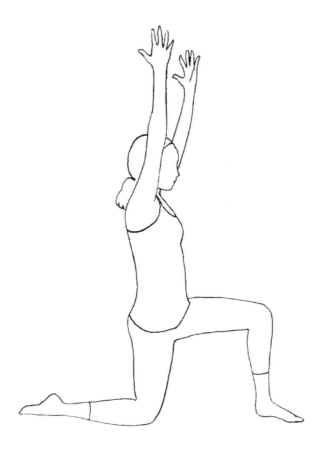

low lunge, staying up and tucking tailbone

In the version shown on this page, the torso is more upright, but the tailbone is tucked very strongly. That creates a psoas stretch that's just as deep. The pose doesn't *look* as deep, but it *feels* just as deep or even deeper – and that's what matters. This is the version I usually recommend for most people, because it provides the release that's actually needed.

How to Protect Your Low Back

- Keep the tailbone tucked when doing backbends of the lower back, using lumbosacral rhythm to prevent hyperextension.
- Keep away from maximal depth in forward bends, to prevent damage to the lumbar discs and the thoracolumbar fascia. The sympathetic nature of the cervical and lumbar curves may help.
- Use caution with asymmetrical poses of the pelvis, as these can damage the SI joints.

Having examined the spine, it's now time to explore the limbs. In the next few chapters, we'll explore how to keep the arms safe during yoga practice. If you're like most people, you've had discomfort in the shoulders or wrists at some point in your yoga practice; the next section will help you understand why, and what to do about it.

SECTION 3:
THE ARMS

Now that we've explored the spine, we'll take a look at the limbs. In this section, we'll explore the arms, from shoulders to hands.

The shoulders are complex and relatively unprotected, and require special consideration to protect them in yoga. Several common poses may cause shoulder soreness if performed incorrectly. The elbows are much simpler joints, but can still experience damage if moved in certain ways. The wrists are a common source of pain for practitioners, particularly in poses like downward-facing dog.

We'll start at the top, with a look at the shoulders.

CHAPTER 8:
THE SHOULDERS

The shoulders are incredibly complex joints. Each shoulder is actually made up of several different joints, which work together to produce movements of the arm relative to the rest of the body.

The health of the shoulders is essential to our ability to function in our daily lives. People with problems with the shoulder often have trouble performing basic tasks, like combing their hair or reaching into a cabinet for a dish.

The shoulders are optimized for mobility, rather than for stability. The shoulders have a wider range of motion than any other joint in the limbs. This enables us easily to reach objects above our heads and to hang by our arms off of a branch, but this mobility also comes with a cost. The shoulders are relatively less protected than are other joints, and are more prone to injury. This is especially true if the body weight is borne on the hands, as is often the case in yoga.

Understanding the structure of the joints that make up the shoulder will help you to protect this important but vulnerable area. Let's start by looking at the bones involved in the shoulder.

Bones of the Shoulders

What we call "the shoulder" is actually several joints that work together in concert to produce the movements of the arm. The upper arm bone (humerus), shoulder blade (scapula), and collarbone (clavicle) are all involved.

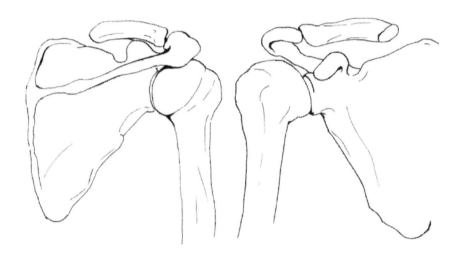

bones of the shoulder; back view on left, front view on right

The upper arm bone, or humerus, is a long bone with a ball at the top. It forms a ball-and-socket joint, within which it can move through a wide range of motion.

But where's the socket? My students often pause for a moment on this one.

The socket of that ball-and-socket joint is in the shoulder blade, or scapula. The head of the humerus sits in a little cup on the side of the scapula called the glenoid fossa. This joint between the glenoid and the humerus is called the glenohumeral joint. This joint is probably what you think of first when you think of the shoulder. While movement at this joint accounts for a large proportion of the arm's range of motion, it's certainly not all of it.

The scapula doesn't form joints with any other bones. It slides around on the back, gliding over thin layers of fat known as the "gliding planes" (because "thin layers of fat" just doesn't sound as good). This is called the scapulothoracic joint, even though it isn't a joint at all; it's just a bone sliding around on soft tissue.

The scapula has a great deal of freedom to move around on the back in its non-joint. It can slide up and down, slide side to side, and rotate on the back. These movements of the scapula contribute significantly to the shoulder's range of motion.

If you feel along the back of your scapula, you'll find a ridge of bone running across it, diagonally up and out. This is the spine of the scapula. (You can see this in the above illustration of the shoulder bones.) Keep following it, and you'll find that it continues outward to form a little point of bone at the outside of your shoulder. That's the acromion (from the same root word as acropolis – think of a platform above a city). It's an important structure, and it needs to be considered to keep the shoulder healthy, as we'll soon explore.

If you keep following the acromion around your shoulder, you'll feel it meet your collarbone, or clavicle. You may be able to feel the little line where the acromion and the clavicle meet. This is the acromioclavicular joint, or AC joint.

The AC joint is a synovial joint, and although its range of movement isn't huge, it's an important part of the movement of the arm. You can feel this by placing your left fingers gently over your right AC joint and then moving your right arm around; you'll feel movement there, perhaps more movement than you expected. If the AC joint is damaged and its range of motion reduced, then the scapula will be restricted as well, and the shoulder correspondingly less mobile.

The clavicle is shaped like an *S*. Follow it towards the center of your body, and you'll feel where it connects to your breastbone, or sternum. This is the sternoclavicular joint, or SC joint. Again, though it feels like there isn't a lot of space there, this is a synovial joint that must move in order to have a healthy shoulder; if you place your fingers over it and move your arm around, you'll feel the small movements occurring there.

To summarize, the shoulder is made up of four joints (one of which isn't actually a joint): the glenohumeral joint, the scapulothoracic joint, the acromioclavicular joint, and the sternoclavicular joint. To have a healthy shoulder, you need all of these joints to be healthy.

It's interesting to think about how loosely connected the arm is to the spine. The weight of the arm is in the humerus; this connects to the scapula, then the clavicle, then the sternum. To find the connection to the spine, you'd need to keep going, from the sternum to the ribs and around to the spine.

Contrast that to the legs. The femur connects to the pelvis, which connects to the spine. There's a more solid connection there. By contrast, the arm is almost dangling in space.

The scapula and the clavicle are part of the "shoulder girdle." They're really arm bones, even though they're on your torso. If you didn't have an arm, you wouldn't need a scapula nor a clavicle. They may at first seem like core bones, but they're actually arm bones.

The Labrum

The head of the humerus is much too large to fit into the glenoid fossa securely. That creates an inherent instability at this joint.

There's a little bit of extra stability in the form of a rim of cartilage that attaches around the edges of the glenoid. This rim is called the labrum (LAY-brum). It makes the socket deeper, so that it can hold the head of the humerus a little bit more securely. It also distributes synovial fluid, and spreads out force within the joint.

The labrum is vulnerable. When movement at the glenohumeral joint reaches the edges of its range of motion, there is compression of the labrum, as the head of the humerus presses into the edges of the glenoid. If this persists, then the labrum (which is made of cartilage) will be slowly worn down. Eventually, it may simply give out and rupture. This is known as a chronic labral tear. It's extremely painful, and it also leaves the shoulder with instability.

Like other cartilage, the labrum has a very poor ability to heal. That's why it's important to be aware of the edges of the glenohumeral joint's range of motion, to ensure that you don't cause damage to the labrum.

When the shoulder is dislocated at the glenohumeral joint, the head of the humerus pops out from the glenoid. As it moves over the labrum, it causes damage. Even after the head of the humerus is put back into its socket, the labrum will remain weaker at the spot where the humerus was forced across it, and the shoulder will be permanently more likely to dislocate again in the same direction.

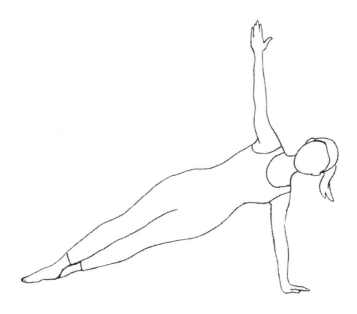

side plank

Because the shoulder is optimized for mobility rather than stability, it's vulnerable to dislocation when bearing the body weight on the hands. For example, during side plank, it's best to keep the shoulder stacked directly over the wrist. This supports the body weight in a stable way. If the shoulder is in front of the wrist, then gravity may cause the yoga practitioner to fall forward, which could dislocate the shoulder. (Having the shoulder behind the wrist is also safe, since the feet are on the floor, preventing the body from suddenly being pulled in that direction.) At the same time, using the muscles of the area to actively hold the shoulder in place is also important.

Another pose that can put the shoulders at risk for dislocation is chaturanga (low plank). The common cue to keep the elbows tucked in next to the ribs is an important one for safety, for the shoulders as well as for the elbows themselves. With the upper arms directly next to the torso, the shoulders are much less wobbly than if the elbows were floated away from the body. Keeping the arms in this position requires a great deal of muscular strength; it's better to keep the shoulders safe and do the pose with the knees on the floor than to keep the knees up and let the elbows migrate away from the body.

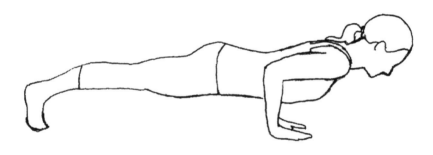

chaturanga

When someone "separates" their shoulder, it means that the

dislocation occurred at the AC joint, rather than at the glenohumeral joint. This takes tremendous force, such as occurs in a car crash or football. The likelihood of separating your shoulder in yoga is extremely close to zero (although you might manage it during acroyoga, a partner balancing practice, if you fell in exactly the wrong way).

Range of Motion

As a ball-and-socket joint, the glenohumeral joint can perform six basic movements. Knowing what to call them will make it easier to discuss each one.

When the arm moves toward the front of the body, it's called flexion. There's a huge range for flexion of the shoulder; in full flexion, the arm is vertical. When the arm moves toward the back of the body, this is extension. (This can seem confusing to some people, because our colloquial language may refer to bringing the arms above the head as "extension," when in scientific terms, this is flexion.)

When the arm is brought out to the side, as in making a snow angel, that's abduction; in adduction, the arm is brought toward (and, in full adduction, across) the midline of the body.

Rotation is also possible at the joint. When an imaginary line on the front of the arm moves toward the outside of the body, that's external rotation; when it moves toward the midline of the body, that's internal rotation. It may be easier to visualize the rotational movements with the elbow flexed (bent). When the hand is pointing straight forward, the shoulder is neutral. When the upper arm rotates so that the hand moves away from the body, that's external rotation of the shoulder; when the rotation brings the hand toward the abdomen, that's internal rotation.

Movements of the scapulothoracic joint are also important. When the scapula glides upward on the body, that's called elevation. When the scapula glides downward, that's called depression. Bringing the scapula outward, toward the side of the body, is known as protraction, while bringing the scapula toward the spine is known as retraction.

Flexion and Extension

The shoulder can flex up to 180° in most people. At this point, the upper arms will be alongside the ears. Many "classic" yoga cues tell students to bring their arms alongside the ears.

However, not all shoulders are shaped exactly the same way. For some, the safe range for flexion is less than 180°. Unfortunately, I too often hear yoga teachers telling students whose shoulders don't flex to a fully vertical position that they have "tight lats," and that if they keep working on it, then they'll get their arms to align next to their ears.

There are some students who truly are limited by muscular tightness in the lats and pecs. For these students, their shoulders may indeed gain the ability to flex to 180° once these muscles become looser. For many others, however, the limitation is not the muscles at all, but the bones. Attempting to get their shoulders to flex farther than they already do will only lead to damage to the labrum and the articular cartilage of the shoulder.

How can someone figure out which type of limitation they have? Recall the tension and compression discussion from Chapter 4. Someone whose shoulder flexion is limited by muscular tightness will feel tension – a pulling or stretching sensation, most likely in the lats (on the back) or pecs (on the chest), as they flex their shoulders. As long as the sensation stays in the belly of the muscle and doesn't migrate toward the joint itself, there's no danger here. The muscles can be stretched, and over time, the tension will release and the shoulder will be freed to reveal its true full range of motion. Of course, that might still be less than 180°, but you can't tell until the muscles are released.

However, if the issue is that the joint has simply reached the end of its range, then the student will feel a pinching or squeezing in the shoulder joint itself. (In my experience, this is far more common than is limitation by tightness of the muscles; admittedly, this is an unscientific observation.) I sometimes hear students say something like, "It feels crowded," or, "It just feels like there's no space in there." This indicates that the end of the safe range of motion for flexion has been reached.

Continuing to try to get more flexion out of this shoulder will damage the joint; the labrum could tear, and the articular cartilage could be worn away. If this continues for years, osteoarthritis of the shoulder could be the result.

Why do the shoulders need to align next to the ears in 180° of flexion? As far as I can tell, the main reason is aesthetics. Completely vertical arms look cleaner and more organized. Other than that, I can't think of a single anatomical reason why shoulders at 170° (for example) wouldn't be just as good. Unfortunately, many students are risking injury trying to achieve that 180° "perfect" form. And just to make a pose prettier? It's not worth it.

I cringe when I hear yoga teachers telling students to keep working on getting their shoulders to flex further. When it's a bony limitation, as it often is, this is a really bad idea. The same idea applies to any movement of the shoulder. When you feel pinching or squeezing in your shoulder joint, that's your body's signal to stop pushing it. If you don't honor the signal, you're hurting yourself. Isn't yoga supposed to be about non-harming?

External and Internal Rotation

When the arm is raised (whether via flexion or abduction), it may be in neutral rotation, or in external or internal rotation. The combination of these movements is crucial to keeping the shoulder healthy for life.

Let's try a little exercise that I use in trainings to demonstrate how important rotation is. Starting with your arm in neutral rotation (i.e., just hanging loosely by your side), begin to move your arm to the side, away from your body, like you're making a snow angel (i.e., abduct your shoulder). Go very slowly, and keep your awareness in your shoulder joint. You'll hit a point where you just don't want to abduct your arm any further; your shoulder starts to feel crowded, and while you could force it to go further, it wouldn't feel good (please don't force it!). For me, it's about 30° above the horizontal plane, but everyone's shoulder is different.

Bring your arm back to your side, releasing the movement. Now, externally rotate your shoulder, so that the imaginary line on the front of your arm moves toward the outside of your body. Keeping your shoulder in external rotation, abduct your arm again, going slowly and feeling for crowding in the shoulder joint.

Almost everyone finds a much greater range of motion with the arm in external rotation. (Of course, all shoulders are different, and occasionally someone can move freely with the arm in neutral rotation. If this is the case for you, and you're a yoga teacher, be aware that most of your students will have more space when in external rotation.)

Why does external rotation give the shoulder a greater range of abduction?

There's a bump on the humerus called the greater tuberosity. Like most bumps on bones, it's the site of attachment of muscles – in this case, two of the powerful rotator cuff muscles. When the arm is in neutral rotation and the arm is abducted, the greater tuberosity presses into the underside of the acromion. That's what causes the feeling of crowding in the shoulder. Externally rotating the shoulder moves this bump out of the way, so that when the arm is abducted, the greater tuberosity is behind the acromion. That way, when the arm is raised, there's no pressure between the two structures. The shoulder feels much more freedom.

Beyond making the shoulder feel better, this action helps to protect an important structure of the shoulder. Under the acromion, there's a bursa, called (somewhat uncreatively) the subacromial bursa. As discussed in Chapter 2, a bursa is a small sac of synovial fluid that protects a tendon from damage from a rough spot on a bone. In this case, the subacromial bursa is there to protect the tendon of one of the rotator cuff muscles, the supraspinatus (soup-ra-spin-AY-tus).

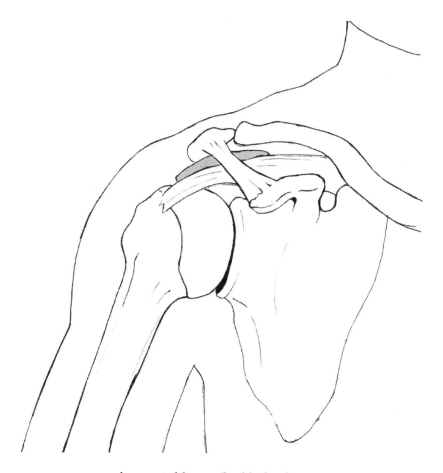

subacromial bursa (highlighted in gray)

When the greater tuberosity presses into the acromion, it squishes that bursa. If this happens repeatedly, the bursa can become inflamed – this is known as bursitis, and it's painful and debilitating on its own. If the inflammation continues, then the structures of the shoulder will start to become damaged and scars will form. Then the shoulder's range of motion is affected. This damage, unfortunately, is often permanent.

It's really important to prevent this situation. Doing so is simple: whenever the shoulder is flexed or abducted, it should also be externally rotated. Every time. I use the horizontal plane as the guide; if the arm comes above the horizontal plane, externally rotate the shoulder. Many

113

people can safely take their arms a little higher, but the horizontal plane is a safe guide to use to protect everyone's shoulders.

Unfortunately, I almost never hear this cue in a yoga class. Equally unfortunately, I often hear yoga students say that certain poses hurt their shoulders – and this is why. I constantly emphasize this one in my teacher trainings and workshops, because most people seem to be unaware of it, and it's so important.

It can get confusing to think about the rotation of the shoulders when they're also in full flexion. When your arms are hanging by your sides and you externally rotate them, your palms face forward. When you then fully flex or abduct your shoulders with them still externally rotated, your palms face *backward*. That's what you want whenever your arms are up above the horizontal plane.

Actually, because the forearms can also be rotated, it works better to look at the "eyes of your elbows" – that soft inner hollow – to figure out the rotation of the shoulder. That's a more direct way to evaluate the shoulder's position, since it's unaffected by what's happening in the forearm. External rotation means that eyes of your elbows face *forward* (and slightly to the outside) when your arms are down, and they face *backward* (still slightly to the outside) when your arms are up. This gets very confusing for many people! If you're ever unsure, you can dissect the movement; bring your arms out of flexion without changing their rotation, and then check how your upper arm is rotated.

The arms come up above horizontal many, many times throughout a yoga practice, and when you first start thinking about this issue, it'll seem like you're constantly adjusting the rotation of your shoulders. For instance, the shoulders are flexed in chair pose (utkatasana) – so they should be externally rotated. This is a pose in which people commonly experience pinching or squeezing in the shoulders, but ignore it because they're focusing on the work they're doing in the legs. A simple rotation of the arms will fix the problem.

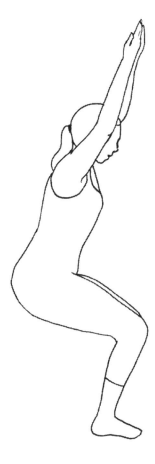

chair pose

Keep in mind that while "face your palms toward the back of the room" is a good first approximation to cue external rotation in flexed shoulders, the cue isn't perfect and won't work for everyone. Using this cue in a pose like chair will result in most people externally rotating their shoulders, but a few may keep the shoulder in neutral or even internal rotation, and supinate (rotate) the forearms.

When the arms are brought above the head during a sun salutation, and then you "swan dive" down to a forward fold (if that's the version you prefer), it's tempting to turn the palms outward as you go down – but don't! That's internal rotation, and your shoulders will not appreciate that action. Instead, leave the palms facing upward until your arms are horizontal, then flip them over if you want to.

In downward-facing dog, the shoulders are fully flexed. (Remember, they may not be next to the ears at full flexion – don't force them there.) That means they should also be externally rotated. In this case, because the body weight is loaded onto the arms, externally rotating the shoulders requires a great deal of effort. You want the eyes of your elbows (that soft inner part) pointing toward the front of your mat (which is behind your back) to the best of your ability.

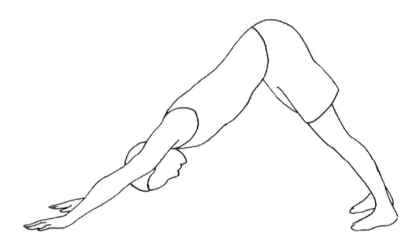

downward dog

At the same time, you're also rotating the forearms to bring the palms to the floor, so there's a lot of muscular strength and coordination required. Keep this in mind if you're teaching a class; don't ask people to stay in downward dog for too long, since they'll need to use so much strength to keep the shoulders externally rotated while pronating the forearms. You don't want them to get tired and start losing their ability to keep the shoulders aligned. (More on pronation in the next chapter.)

If you're one of the many students who find that down dog hurts their shoulders, then this is likely to help you. I've unfortunately heard people say that they quit doing yoga because this very common pose was painful for their shoulders (or their wrists, which we'll get to in a couple of chapters). Giving up the many benefits of yoga, when a simple arm rotation could have helped – what a tragedy!

The Rotator Cuff

Because it's optimized for mobility, there are very few ligaments stabilizing the shoulder. The joint capsule of the shoulder is relatively thin and weak, and there's not much connective tissue holding the head of the humerus into the glenoid.

To make up for this lack of ligamentous stability, the shoulder is stabilized by a group of muscles known as the rotator cuff. They're often referred to as "active ligaments," because these muscles serve the same functions that ligaments serve in other joints; namely, to stabilize the joint and keep it from being dislocated.

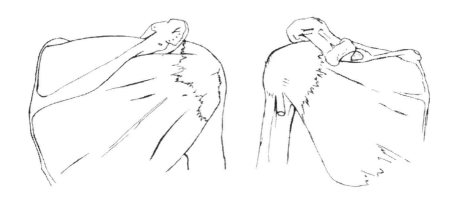

rotator cuff; back view on left, front view on right

These four muscles originate on the scapula itself, forming a coating of muscle on the scapula on both the front and back. They cross the glenohumeral joint and attach to the head of the humerus (two of them attach at the greater tuberosity, that bony bump that causes the problem with the subacromial bursa if it's not moved out of the way). As you can see in the illustration, the tendons of the rotator cuff muscles look very much like a group of ligaments stabilizing the humerus in the scapula – and that's essentially what they are.

The actions of the rotator cuff muscles are complementary to each other. Two externally rotate the arm, one internally rotates it, and the last one abducts it. When they're all contracted at the same time, the humerus is held in place and prevented from slipping out of the glenoid. (The muscle that performs abduction is able to hold the arm up so that gravity doesn't pull it downward out of the socket – a particularly important action when holding a heavy object.)

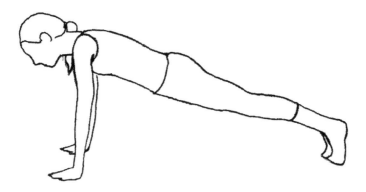

plank pose

When bearing the body weight on the hands – even just part of the body weight, like in plank – it's necessary to actively engage these muscles to ensure the stability of the shoulder. Remember that the shoulder isn't optimized for bearing weight, so you have to consciously create the required stability to allow you to do that. I find that cues like "hug your arm bones into their sockets" are helpful. You'll feel a muscular engagement along the front and back of your scapula when your rotator cuff is engaged. Your goal is to create this engagement any time you're bearing weight on your hands. It's most crucial when bearing all of your body weight there, such as in handstand, but is still important in poses like plank and side plank.

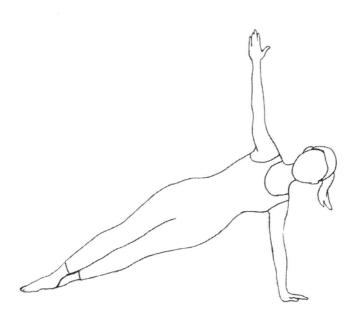

side plank

The Traps

The trapezius muscle (commonly known as "the trap") consists of three parts: upper, middle, and lower. It attaches all along the cervical and upper thoracic spine, and attaches to the scapula. The upper part of the trapezius elevates the scapula (pulls it upward), while the lower part depresses it (pulls it downward). That makes these two parts of a single muscle antagonists of each other.

When you're hunching your shoulders, your upper traps are engaged. They're also working when you carry weight on top of your shoulder, such as a backpack or purse. Because most of us do both of these things frequently, almost everyone has overdeveloped upper traps.

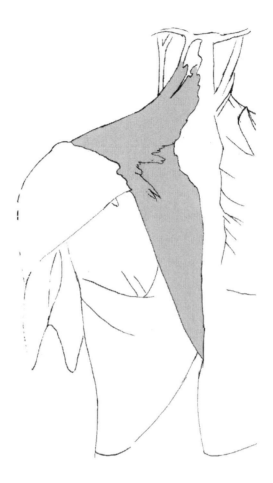

trapezius (highlighted in gray)

Recall from Chapter 3 that reciprocal inhibition causes muscles that are antagonists to inhibit each other when they contract. Reciprocal inhibition causes the lower traps to be relaxed whenever the upper traps are working, because these two are antagonists of each other. Because the upper traps are often so tight, the lower traps are usually weak and floppy.

Many people feel discomfort in their upper traps and want to relieve it. Sometimes, people do this by stretching the upper traps. Bringing the arm back and down behind you, then leaning your head in the opposite direction, will accomplish this. (Use caution, because sometimes this pose stretches the nerves of the arm, leading to tingling in the fingers; if this happens, release the arm forward.) While the stretch feels nice, there's a better way to relax the upper traps. You can use reciprocal inhibition in your favor.

Pulling your shoulder blades down your back activates the lower traps. By reflex, the upper traps will soften. The more you draw your shoulder blades down your back, the softer your upper traps will get. At first, because the lower traps are weak and infrequently activated, using them will feel very strange, and you may feel like they fatigue quickly. Like any muscle, they'll get stronger with use, and strengthening them will help soften a problematic area of muscle tension. So keep working on them. You'll be glad that you did.

How To Protect Your Shoulders

- Never force your shoulders to move into a range where they feel pinched or squeezed, to protect the labrum and cartilage.
- When bearing weight on the hands, ensure that there is as little wobbling as possible. Keep the shoulder over the wrist in plank and side plank, and elbows tucked next to the body in chaturanga, to protect the shoulders.
- Always externally rotate your shoulders when they come above the horizontal plane, to prevent impingement of the subacromial bursa.
- Keep your muscles engaged, with arm bones hugging into their sockets, whenever you're bearing weight on the hands, to prevent shoulder dislocation.

While the shoulder is inherently unstable, the elbow is a very stable joint. In the next chapter, we'll look at the true elbow joint as well as the joint that allows the forearm to rotate, which is a separate joint. Let's move down the arm to explore the elbow.

CHAPTER 9:
THE ELBOWS

In contrast to the shoulder, the elbow is a very stable joint protected by many ligaments. Osteoarthritis in the elbow is less common than the same problem in other, less stable joints, such as the shoulder or knee. However, compression of the ulnar nerve at the elbow, known as cubital tunnel syndrome, is relatively common, and can be caused or exacerbated by a yoga practice.

The elbow gets a lot of attention in certain yoga traditions, as many teachers have been taught to be concerned about "hyperextension" of the elbow joint. We'll discuss later why this concern may be misplaced.

Let's start by exploring the bones and joints that make up the elbow.

Bones

We looked at the upper part of the humerus in the previous chapter. Near the elbow, the humerus widens. Those two bumps you feel on either side of your elbow are part of the humerus. Between them is a hollow called the olecranon (oh-LECK-rah-non) fossa.

There are two bones in the forearm: the ulna and the radius. The ulna is wide towards the elbow, and narrow towards the wrist. The bony "point" of your elbow is part of your ulna; specifically, it's the olecranon process. When the elbow extends (straightens), the olecranon process fits into the olecranon fossa. This joint between the humerus and the ulna is the true elbow joint. In the illustration below, you can see the olecranon process fitting securely into the olecranon fossa. (The ulna is the bone on the lower left, and the humerus is on top.)

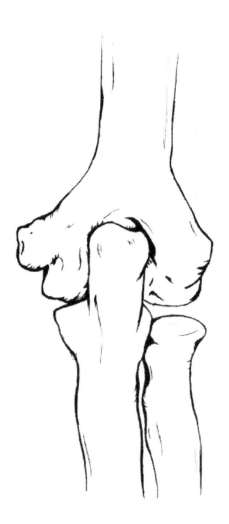

straight elbow viewed from behind; ulna fitting into humerus

The elbow joint has a thick capsule, and is also protected by many ligaments along the sides of the joint. These are known as the collateral ligaments. Given the highly congruent bony anatomy and the abundant connective tissue, this is one of the most stable joints in the body.

The radius is narrow towards the elbow and wide towards the wrist. It forms most of the wrist joint; we'll look more at that in the next chapter. Near the elbow, the radius ends in a small cylindrical piece. You can see this toward the right in the illustration above. This cylinder rests against the ulna and rolls around it as the forearm rotates. This joint between the radius and the ulna is separate from the joint between the humerus and the ulna, with a separate joint capsule.

The radius is held to the ulna with the annular ligament. "Annulus" is Latin for "ring," which tells you how this ligament is shaped. The annular ligament comes from the ulna, passes around the radius, and inserts back onto the ulna, forming a sling around the radius that holds it in place but allows it to roll.

Range of Motion

The elbow joint itself (the joint between the humerus and the ulna) can only flex (bend) and extend (straighten). Because of the abundance of ligaments on both sides of the elbow (the collateral ligaments), any side-to-side or rotational movement is prevented at this joint. (This is quite different from the knee joint, as we'll see in Chapter 12.)

At the radioulnar joint, the radius rolls around the ulna. As this joint moves, the forearm is rotated. The movements are referred to as pronation and supination. With your elbow by your side and flexed to about 90°, flip your palm upward; this is supination. (I was taught to remember it as "supination is like carrying a bowl of soup.") Now flip your palm down; this is pronation. (You can think of this as…"pouring out your soup.")

Flexion and Extension

The strong collateral ligaments that prevent lateral or rotational movement of the ulna on the humerus are important in protecting this joint. As long as these ligaments stay healthy, the joint is very stable, and can only move in one plane.

Although it doesn't come up very frequently, it's not a good idea to put sideways pressure onto the elbow, or any pressure that would attempt to rotate the arm at the humeroulnar joint. In some forms of yoga, arm poses like "pigeon for the arm" are used, which put pressure on the arm in an attempt to cause rotation of the lower arm on the upper arm (similar to the rotation that's possible at the knee). These poses have the potential to cause damage to the cartilage of this joint, because rotation at the elbow is not possible; additionally, they can damage the ligaments that support the joint. Use caution if you decide to do these poses, and be aware that the elbow joint is actually incapable of rotation so that you don't try to force it into potentially damaging positions.

The Ulnar Nerve

There are three main nerves that supply the forearm and hand with sensation and motor control: the ulnar, median, and radial nerves. The ulnar nerve's path takes it alongside the olecranon process, just inside that bump on the humerus, on the pinky-finger side of the arm.

In this position, the ulnar nerve is very poorly protected. When that area gets hit, an electrical zapping or tingling feeling goes down your forearm and into your pinky finger; this is often referred to as "bumping your funny bone."

The ulnar nerve travels through a little tunnel of connective tissue as it makes its way through the elbow. This is called the cubital tunnel. If there's inflammation in this tissue, the space for the nerve is reduced, and the nerve may get compressed. In this case, people will experience that sensation of tingling in the pinky finger (often along with part of the ring finger and the side of the hand) frequently or continuously. If it's not addressed, numbness of the pinky-finger side of the hand can occur, followed by weakness of the muscles served by the ulnar nerve (including certain muscles that control the hand).

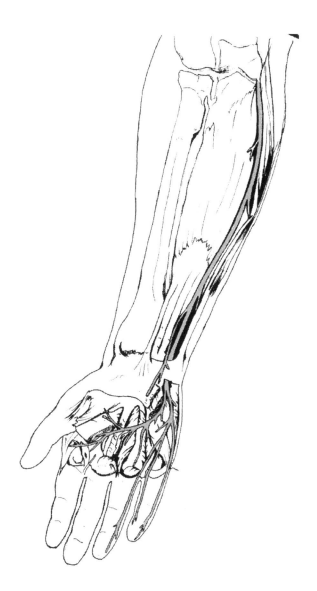

ulnar nerve (highlighted in gray)

If you feel tingling in your pinky finger, it's definitely worth addressing it before it progresses. The swelling of the connective tissue and compression of the nerve can be a result of overuse of the elbow; this is often referred to as "tennis elbow," but it doesn't just occur with tennis. This injury can occur with any activity that repeatedly and forcefully flexes and extends the elbow. An example in yoga is doing chaturanga over and over, which is incredibly common in yoga classes (think about how many times you hear "take a vinyasa" in a typical flow class).

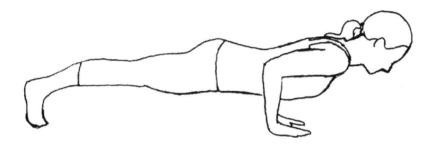

chaturanga

Chaturanga is particularly likely to injure the elbow if it's performed with the elbows held out to the sides, rather than next to the body. This puts uneven stress on the inside and outside of the elbow joint, potentially causing damage to the tendons and ligaments. If this inflammation affects the cubital tunnel, then the ulnar nerve may become compressed. Besides protecting the shoulders, which it also does, keeping the elbows right next to the body protects them. (However, even well-aligned chaturangas can still cause tennis elbow if you do too many of them.)

If you find your pinky finger tingling after a class where you did lots of chaturanga, please honor this signal from your body. During class, when your elbow starts to feel sore or your finger starts to tingle, stop doing chaturanga for that day. Immediately. Even with your knees down. Just skip those "optional vinyasas," even if your neighbor is still doing them and you're afraid that you'll look like a quitter. You don't win yoga class by doing the most chaturangas. You win yoga class by having your body feel great afterward.

If the tingling happens frequently, doesn't go away, or gets worse, you should address it with your doctor. This book can help you to avoid causing this injury in yoga, but isn't intended to address how to treat it once it occurs. (Of course, I can never promise the prevention of any medical problem, including this one. The human body, and your life in yours, is simply too complex to make that promise. I can only help you have the safest possible yoga practice.)

Pronation and Supination

In yoga, pronation and supination are generally used to position the hand to contact the ground or another surface. There aren't really particular poses that are targeted to working on these movements.

In some cases, pronation and supination can cause confusion; the ability of the forearm to rotate is the reason that you can't reliably use the position of the hand to determine whether the shoulder is externally or internally rotated. Most commonly, external rotation of the shoulder while the arms are up points the palms backward. However, you could externally rotate and fully flex the shoulder, and then pronate your forearm so that your palm faces forward.

Try it now: externally rotate and flex your shoulder, then hold the elbow steady with your other hand as you turn your palm to face forward. As we discussed in Chapter 8, this is the ideal position of the arms in downward-facing dog, although maintaining it while part of the body weight is loaded onto the hands takes a great deal of muscular strength.

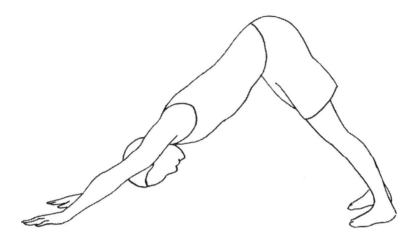

downward dog

The annular ligament is important in holding the radius securely on the ulna as it rolls around it during pronation and supination. If you're carrying weight, this ligament is at risk of being overstretched if the forearm is pronated and the elbow is flexed. (If you flex your elbow to 90° and then turn your palm to the ground, you'll be in this position. Many people use this arm position when carrying things.)

While it may not come up much during a yoga practice, many yoga teachers and even students carry a fair amount of stuff around a yoga studio. Ideally, to protect your annular ligament, it's best to carry things with the forearm supinated, rather than pronated. This means that when you bend your elbow, your palm should be pointing upward while carrying things. As a bonus, the biceps brachii (the big muscle of the upper arm, which flexes the elbow) is strongest when the forearm is supinated, so you can carry heavy objects a little more easily in this position.

The radius can also be dislocated out of the annular ligament by a sharp tug on the forearm. This is sometimes referred to as "nursemaid's elbow." This also doesn't really come up in yoga, but it's a good reason to avoid swinging your kids around by the arms. They do love it, but their elbows are at risk; at the very least, hold both of their hands instead of swinging them by just one.

"Hyperextension"

For most people, the elbow extends (straightens) to about 180° (a straight line). It may be a little more, or it may be a little less. For some reason, although those who have a range of motion of less than 180° are usually not bothered about it, those with a range of motion of greater than 180° are told that they're "hyperextending" and they should stop it.

Medically, hyperextension refers to taking a joint beyond its natural range of extension, into the zone of potential damage. For some people, their natural range of extension is past 180°. This is actually not called hyperextension; rather, the term for this is recurvation. For those with recurvation of the elbows, bringing them into their full extension is not necessarily damaging. An elbow experiencing hyperextension would have that crowded compression sensation; an elbow that recurves but is still in a safe range will not feel compressed.

There are, as previously mentioned, hypermobility syndromes that can lead to joints moving in unsafe ways because they're not protected adequately. However, forcing the elbow into excessive extension is generally not among the problems encountered by hypermobile yoga students. Hypermobile people frequently damage hips and shoulders; but elbows, usually not. Ironically, the elbow seems to be the only joint that many yoga teachers are worried about.

It seems that yoga teachers view an elbow that extends past 180° as a sign that a student is hypermobile. However, these two conditions are unrelated. A student with very tight connective tissue can easily have an elbow that extends past horizontal, while a student with very loose connective tissue (true hypermobility) may not extend this far. The range of elbow extension is not determined solely by ligaments, but by the olecranon of the elbow fitting into its fossa. Whether your connective tissue is loose or tight doesn't really matter; it's the shape of your bones that determines how far your elbow will extend. As with most joints, there's individual variability in the shapes of the bones at the elbow.

In other words, while hypermobility is an issue to be concerned about, it can't be diagnosed based on the elbow's ability to extend. For some reason, yoga appears to have decided to figure how who's hypermobile based on this unreliable sign, yet continues to celebrate those who do transversal splits (which is much more likely to be a sign of hypermobility).

Here's a case of yoga teachers actually overprotecting, rather than underprotecting, their students. Those with elbows that extend a little farther than 180° are usually told to "microbend" their elbows to keep them at 180°. In many cases, this actually isn't necessary.

The only anatomical argument in favor of a microbend is that microbending ensures that muscular strength is contributing to holding up the weight of the body, putting a smaller load on the joints (including the elbow). If this is the reason for the microbend, then everyone should be microbending, whatever their natural range of extension may be. Don't discriminate by asking only those with elbows slightly past the arbitrary cutoff of 180° to microbend, and allowing those with elbows that bend slightly less than 180° to hang out at the end of their range. If you sense that enough body weight is on the elbow that it could be damaging to the articular cartilage to lock out the joint, then you should be using a microbend regardless of the elbow's angle.

Keep in mind that putting that slight bend in the elbow requires a great deal more muscular effort than does locking out the elbow. Therefore, if you're teaching a yoga class and you ask people to microbend their elbows, they're not going to be able to stay in the pose as long as they would if their elbows were locked. That's not necessarily a problem; building strength is a good thing. Just remember that microbending will make poses harder, and that you may want to consider that when planning how long you ask people to stay in the pose.

The belief that recurvation of the elbows is a sign of hypermobility could also be damaging to students who are truly hypermobile. If they hear another student being told that they're hypermobile based on their elbows going past 180°, and the hypermobile student's own elbows stop at or before the horizontal, then the hypermobile student may falsely believe that he or she isn't hypermobile because of elbow shape.

It's not necessary to be particularly concerned about people's elbows extending past 180°. There are far more important things to be concerned about during yoga practice.

How To Protect Your Elbows

- Don't put any sideways pressure on the elbow joint, to protect its articular cartilage.
- Be aware of the potential for overuse syndromes when you do repetitive movements like chaturanga. Limit the number of times you do the same movement in a single yoga session, to protect the ulnar nerve.
- Keep the forearm in a supinated position when lifting objects, to protect the annular ligament of the radius.
- It's okay for your elbow to be beyond 180°, as long as there's no pain or feeling of compression in the joint. If you choose to do a microbend of the elbows, do so regardless of the angle of your extended elbow.

In the next chapter, we'll move down from the elbows to explore the wrists and hands. Wrist pain in yoga is quite common, and traditional alignment cues often do little to relieve the problem. If you've had wrist pain in poses like downward-facing dog, or if you know someone who has, the next chapter may help you adjust your practice to be healthier for your wrists.

CHAPTER 10:
THE WRISTS AND HANDS

The wrist is an unfortunate source of pain for many yoga practitioners. I once taught an entire private yoga session focused on the student's wrist pain. She had believed that she couldn't do yoga because it hurt her wrists. She finally agreed to the private yoga at the insistence of her daughter, whose own yoga practice had provided her too many benefits to allow her to see her mom give up so easily.

Unfortunately, hers is not an uncommon story, and not everyone is lucky enough to have a family member convince them to seek a private yoga teacher to help them fix the wrist issue. Some people give up on yoga entirely because it hurts their wrists.

If you've ever had wrist pain in poses like downward dog, this chapter will help you figure out why, and (more importantly) how to practice without wrist pain.

Bones

As discussed in the previous chapter, there are two bones in the forearm: the radius and the ulna. The ulna is big at the elbow and small at the wrist, while the radius is small at the elbow and big at the wrist.

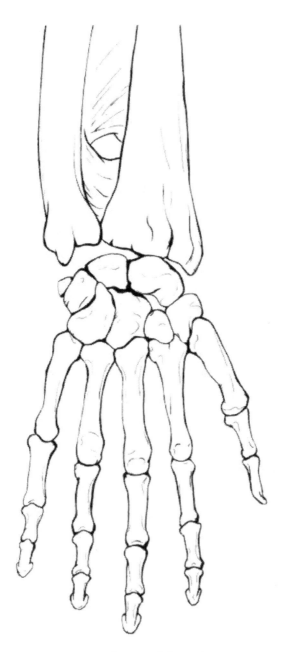

bones of the wrist

Near the wrist, each of the two bones has a little projection of bone sticking out toward the hand. Each projection is called the stylus process. (Anatomists centuries ago probably chose this terminology because giving two different structures the same name makes things more confusing.) The two stylus processes stick up beside the wrist and limit its ability to move side-to-side.

The carpals are often referred to as the "wrist bones," although they're actually located in the heel of the hand. There are eight of them, all small and square-ish. They're bound together by thick connective tissue, into an arch-shaped structure. Feel the heel of your hand, and you'll find this arch. While there are synovial joints between the carpals, and they're capable of gliding movements, the thick connective tissue prevents excessive movement between them. However, the arch of the hand can flatten to absorb force and spring back up to release it. (This is similar to the arch of the foot, which we'll discuss in Chapter 13.)

The radius makes an ellipsoid joint with the first three carpals. Imagine an oval-shaped structure fitting into an oval-shaped cup. The result is that the wrist can flex (bend) and extend (straighten), and can move from side to side, but can't rotate relative to the forearm.

Because the metacarpals (the "rays" of your hand) originate from the carpals, they too have an arch-shaped arrangement, meaning that the entire hand is an arch. This means that the hand doesn't press completely flat into the floor; there will always be a small part of it that's held off the floor. There's no need to attempt to make it flat, as the arch keeps the hand both stable and healthy.

The phalanges (fah-LAN-jeez), or finger bones, come straight from the metacarpals. There are three phalanges in each finger, except that there are only two in the thumb.

Range of Motion

The wrist joint can flex (bend so the palm comes toward your arm) and extend (bend so that the top of your hand comes toward your arm).

In general, flexion has a larger range of motion than does extension.

In addition to flexion and extension, the wrist can also perform abduction and adduction. In most joints, abduction brings the limb away from the body, and adduction brings it toward the midline; however, because position of the shoulder and forearm determines the orientation of the wrist, defining side-to-side movements of the wrist in this way tends to create confusion. That's why other names are usually used for these movements: radial deviation and ulnar deviation.

Holding your arm out in front of you with your wrist flat, bring your hand toward the thumb side (this is called radial deviation, because the hand is moving toward the radius). Then bring your hand toward the pinky finger side (this is ulnar deviation, as you move the hand toward the ulna).

You may notice that you have a greater range of motion for movement toward the thumb side than toward the pinky finger side; that's because the stylus process of the radius is not as long as that of the ulna. If you want to compare them, line up both forearms and hands in front of you, with both palms facing toward you. Bend both wrists to your left, and then to your right; you'll notice that whichever hand is in ulnar deviation can go farther than the one in radial deviation.

The fingers have similar ranges of motion: they can flex (curl) and extend (straighten), and can abduct (spread apart from each other) and adduct (come together), but cannot rotate on their bases. You can draw a circle in the air using a finger, which is called circumduction; however, you can't rotate your finger so that your fingernail faces toward your palm.

The Carpal Tunnel

Across the arch formed by the carpals, there's a piece of connective tissue called the flexor retinaculum. There's a little tunnel between this tissue and the arch of the carpals; it's called the carpal tunnel. Through the tunnel, several important structures pass. One of them is the median nerve, which provides sensation to the middle part of the hand and fingers.

Swelling in this region can cause the median nerve to be compressed. This is known as carpal tunnel syndrome. It causes the typical symptoms of nerve compression, as described in Chapter 4: tingling in the middle part of the hand, followed by numbness in that region, followed by weakness of the hand muscles served by the nerve. This is the most common syndrome of nerve compression in the arm; cubital tunnel syndrome, in which the ulnar nerve is compressed near the elbow, is the second most common. (Cubital tunnel syndrome was discussed in Chapter 9.)

Deep flexion of the wrist causes pressure on the carpal tunnel and the structures within it. That's why many people with carpal tunnel syndrome wake up with tingling fingers; it's very common to sleep with the wrists in deep flexion (unconsciously, of course). Bringing the wrists into deep flexion to check for tingling is actually used as a diagnostic test for carpal tunnel.

It's rare for yoga poses to include very deep wrist flexion; in fact, there aren't many poses that involve flexion at all. However, if you have carpal tunnel syndrome or if you notice that your fingers tingle during this movement, then it's best for you to avoid deep wrist flexion if it does come up.

Wrist extension can also exacerbate carpal tunnel syndrome, by increasing the pressure within the carpal tunnel. That can make it hard for those with carpal tunnel to perform even simple poses on all fours. Extension of the wrist can also be a problem for the wrist joint itself, so even if there is no nerve compression, it's useful to be aware of the limitations of this movement.

Wrist Extension

Extension of the wrist brings the back of the hand toward the forearm. The range of this motion varies between different people, but around 70° is average.

Many yoga poses require 90° of extension. For some people, this is greater than their range. Yoga teachers may teach students to "work on their wrist flexibility" in order to attain a 90° range. However, as we've seen in other joints, that's not the way it works. If you feel compression in your wrist when you extend it to a 90° angle, then the safe range of motion in your wrist won't change when you attempt to force it to.

Even a simple pose like being on all fours (on your hands and knees) may require your wrists to be at or close to 90° of extension, so what's a yogi to do? A simple modification can fix the problem for many students. Just fold a towel or blanket and put it under the heels of your hands, with the base of your fingers off the towel. If you don't have a towel or blanket, or if getting it ready during class interrupts your flow, then folding over the front of your mat and putting the base of your fingers off of it, with the heels of your hands on, will also work.

That modification will place your wrists in a smaller degree of extension. You can fold the towel or your mat to be as tall as you need it to be, until your wrists are comfortable in the pose. Downward dog requires significantly less extension in the wrists and is usually not a problem from this perspective, although if you're doing a vinyasa flow class, you may want to keep the heels of your hands elevated as you flow between plank and downward dog.

Another way to keep your wrists from entering excessive extension is to bear weight primarily at the base of your fingers, so there's less weight pressing the heel of your hand down into the floor. To do this, think of pressing actively through your fingers. The difference it makes is small, but can be meaningful in keeping the wrists healthy. You can also bend your elbows slightly to decrease the amount of wrist extension that's required by the pose.

It's important to practice any pose that requires weight-bearing on the hands on a firm, rather than a soft, surface. Soft surfaces collapse unevenly, with the heels of the hands pressing deeper than the fingers, meaning that the wrist is brought into excessive extension. Further, the squishiness of the surface will make it difficult to balance in an inversion or arm balance, which could make you more likely to fall. This is why yoga mats are generally relatively firm. Some yoga students may practice on a Pilates-style mat, which is about an inch thick and is much softer than a standard yoga mat; if you're going to bear any weight on the hands, which you are almost certain to do in a yoga class unless it's a restorative class, then you're better off with a firmer mat. Similarly, don't practice handstands or arm balances on your carpeted floor, which is usually too soft.

Orienting Your Fingers

When one of the stylus processes presses into the side of the carpals, then it often causes pain in the wrist. This can be the source of discomfort in poses like downward dog.

There are a variety of yogic schools of thought on exactly how the hands should be oriented in downward dog. I've heard the following asserted as the right way to do this: the index fingers must be pointing directly forward, the middle fingers must be pointing directly forward, and the line between the index and middle fingers must be pointing directly forward. Those who subscribe to one of these rules usually seem very committed to their rule as the only way to do the pose correctly, asserting that it's the "proper alignment."

I'd like to discard all this dogma and create a new rule. In downward dog, point your fingers in whichever direction is necessary to make your wrists feel good. If you find that your wrists are sore in this pose, then you may find that adjusting the direction of your fingers brings relief.

I sometimes use the benchmark of the crease that forms at your wrists when you extend them; making this crease parallel to the top of your mat often feels right. However, that's just a starting point. Feel free to modify the direction of your hands in any way you need to, so that your wrists feel spacious in the pose. If anyone dogmatically asserts that you're doing it wrong, the best course of action is to respectfully ignore their (presumably well-intentioned) advice and keep doing it the way that feels right for you.

Muscles of the Hand

Many of the muscles that move the hand are located in the forearm. Feel your forearm as you curl and open your fingers; you'll find those muscles. They're known as the extrinsic muscles of the hand.

Those who spend their days gripping objects may find that there's tightness in these forearm muscles. Releasing the tension in these muscles often feels wonderful. Any pose that brings the wrist into extension will do it. I like to come on all fours with weight more in the knees than the hands, then flip the hands around, so that the fingers are pointing towards me rather than away. Then I sit back slightly toward my heels. This brings the wrist into extension and stretches the forearm muscles. My students love this, although it's important to be aware of the potential for too much wrist extension; cue everyone to feel for wrist compression, and release the pose as necessary to avoid that squeezing sensation.

Because they begin in the forearm and then cross the wrist as well as the finger joints, the extrinsic muscles of the hand are also muscles of the wrist. The effect of this is that the position of the wrist affects the position of the fingers, especially near the ends of the range of motion.

Make a fist. You'll almost certainly find that you can close your fingers tightly. Now, open your hand again. Next, flex (bend) your wrist, so that your palm comes toward your forearm. Go as far as it's comfortable. Then try to make a fist. Much harder, yes?

This happens because the tendons that extend the wrist and fingers are stretched as the wrist is flexed, and begin to pull the fingers slightly into extension when flexion is deep. (Incidentally, martial artists use this technique to force an opponent to drop a weapon; by pressing the opponent's wrist into flexion, the fingers will become incapable of flexing strongly enough to fully grip, no matter how strong the muscles are.)

The converse happens when the wrist is extended. With the wrists flat, extend your fingers back as far as it's comfortable. (That's not very far, usually, but the fingers can come slightly behind the plane of the hand.) Next, extend your wrist by bringing the back of your hand toward your forearm. Notice that your fingers flex (curl) slightly as your wrist comes into full extension.

This comes into play during poses like handstand. The wrist will usually be near the end of its range of motion for extension in this pose. Because of that, the fingers will be pulled by their tendons into slight flexion. You'll feel the pads of your fingers pressing into the mat. Yoga teachers often make a very big deal about it if your fingers are curled slightly, but some students can't help it; it's a tendon thing. (Don't let your fingers curl out of laziness; continue to actively press your fingers into the mat, which will help you balance and will also help spread out the weight of the pose. However, they may curl slightly even while you're doing this.)

How To Protect Your Wrists and Hands

- Watch out for extension (bringing the back of the hand toward the forearm); its range of motion may be less than 90°. If necessary, elevate the heel of the hand on a towel or folded yoga mat, to prevent compression of the wrist.
- In downward dog or other poses that put body weight on the hands, orient the fingers however is necessary to avoid compression in the wrists, to prevent the stylus processes of the radius and ulna from impinging on the carpal bones.
- Don't flex (bend) the wrists deeply if you have carpal tunnel syndrome, or if this motion causes tingling in your hand or fingers.
- Be aware that wrist extension causes slight finger flexion (curling). If you experience this even while actively pressing

through your fingers, don't try to force the fingers into deeper extension, to protect the tendons of the extrinsic muscles of the hand.

Now that we've finished exploring the arm, it's time to move on to the leg. In the next section, we'll finish our exploration of the body with a look at the leg. If you've ever had knee pain in pigeon pose, struggled to "open your hips," or wondered why your ankles are sore in virasana, this next section will help you figure out the problem – and how to protect yourself.

SECTION 4:
THE LEGS

In this section, we'll complete our exploration of the body by learning about the legs, from hips to feet.

The hips are frequently targeted for stretching in yoga classes. They're also one of the most mysterious joints to most people, which leaves them vulnerable to being harmed in a wide variety of poses. The knees are relatively unprotected and unstable joints, but because they bear the body weight, mindful consideration is required to prevent the knees from degenerating. The ankles are more stable, although the feet (particularly their arches) should be carefully attended to throughout a yoga practice.

To begin, let's explore the hips.

CHAPTER 11:
THE HIPS

Yoga practitioners love to "open their hips." It seems like everyone has tight hips – probably because we've spent most of our lives sitting in chairs, at least in most modern societies. Many yoga classes are hip-focused, and nearly every class includes hip openers.

In general, the hip joint is optimized for stability, rather than for mobility. While the hip and the shoulder are both ball-and-socket joints, the hip is quite different from the shoulder in many ways. The socket of the hip is in the solid and stable pelvis, rather than in the smaller and freely mobile scapula (as in the shoulder). The bones have a tighter fit in the hip, and there's plenty of connective tissue supporting the joint.

Because of these structural features, as we're working on "opening our hips" in yoga class, the hips themselves could be said to be resisting this action, working to keep themselves stable. The key is to optimize our range of motion without compromising the stability that we need to keep our hips healthy and functional for life.

Despite the focus on the hips, few yoga practitioners have a good understanding of this joint. It's somewhat hidden, and so it's hard to visualize; most people aren't even certain where the hip joint itself is actually located.

Hip replacements are not uncommon. In fact, they're one of the most common joint replacement surgeries performed. Orthopedic surgeons have reported that they're doing more hip replacements in women who do yoga, quite a few of whom are young (in their 50s or even younger). So we know that protecting the hips is crucial, and it appears that most people don't understand their hips well enough to do that. How can we fix this problem?

Where is the Hip Joint?

If I ask a room full of people to point to their hips, most of them point to their iliac crests (the curves of bone at the top of the pelvis) or to their greater trochanters (the bumps of bone on the upper outer legs). When yoga students are asked to stand with their feet "hip width apart," almost all of them line up the outer edges of their feet with the outer edges of their legs, believing the greater trochanters to be the hips. Standing like this won't hurt you, but "hip width apart" would actually align the feet directly below the hip joints, which are located more toward the center of the body.

The actual hip joint itself is located near the front of the body, in what you might call the groin. In this illustration, take a look at where the femur (thighbone) meets the pelvis, and consider where you would find that joint on your own body.

This knowledge is key, because when you're trying to figure out whether a pose is pinching, squeezing, or otherwise hurting your hips, you need to know where to feel for that sensation. When you're damaging your hip joint, the discomfort won't occur on your outer legs or on the side of your pelvis; it will be in your groin.

The hip joints are structurally not very complicated. Each hip is a ball-and-socket joint, with the ball being the head of the femur (the thighbone) and the socket being a little cup on the pelvis. Let's explore these structures.

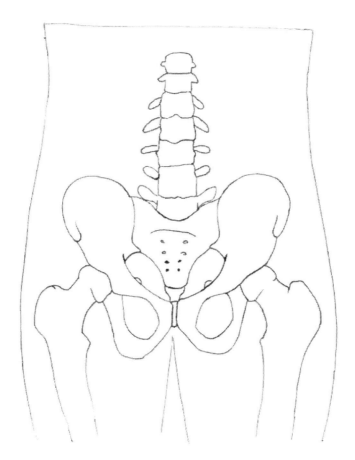

location of the hip joint

The Femur

By virtually any measure, the femur (FEE-mur) is the largest bone in the body. It's the heaviest, and the longest, and the strongest.

The top of the femur ends in a ball, called the head of the femur. Next, there's a thin piece called the neck of the femur. This travels out toward the side of your thigh, toward the bony bump you can feel near the top of your leg on the side. That bump is called the greater trochanter (troh-CANT-er).

At the greater trochanter, the femur makes a turn and then angles down and slightly inward. This part of the femur is variously known as the body or the shaft. Toward the knee, the femur spreads out into two more balls (to be discussed in the next chapter).

There are several angles involved in the anatomy of the femur, and each one varies between individuals. These variations have a major impact on the range of motion of the joint, because they determine the point at which bone will press into bone during various movements of the hip.

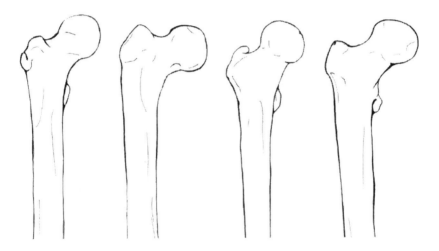

images of several different femurs

For instance, the femoral neck may be longer or shorter, and may also be thinner or wider. A longer and thinner femoral neck provides a greater range of motion, particularly for external rotation and abduction.

The angle made between the body and the neck of the femur also has an impact. Those with a wider angle have a greater range of abduction.

The neck of the femur is also angled forward from the greater trochanter, anywhere from 10° to 30° in most people. Those with a larger forward angle have a smaller range of external rotation, and may feel instability in the hip joint during external rotation, as the head of the femur is pushed forward out of the socket.

Looking at the different femurs above, it's easy to see that expecting them all to behave the same is potentially dangerous. Why would these differently shaped bones all create the exact same movements within the body? As you're performing hip-related yoga poses, you may find it useful to picture your hip joint. Be curious about the shape of your femur, using your experiences in yoga poses as clues. Although it's hard for many of us, conditioned in a competitive world, to avoid comparing ourselves to others in yoga class, it may help to recognize that your bones have their own unique shapes, creating your own unique ideal shape for each pose. You don't win yoga class by having the most external rotation in pigeon. You win yoga class by still being there, with your own natural and pain-free hip joints, in your 80s.

Acetabulum

The head of the femur fits into a socket on the pelvis called the acetabulum (ass-uh-TAB-you-lum).

The fit between these two bones is much more secure than is the fit between the head of the humerus and the glenoid. The acetabulum is deeper than the glenoid, so the amount of contact surface between the ball and the socket is much greater in the hip than in the shoulder. This increased contact between the two bones gives the hip more stability, and also a reduced range of motion compared to the shoulder.

To ensure the stability of the joint, a ligament connects the center of the acetabulum to the head of the femur. (You can see the ends of this ligament on the illustration below.) Within this ligament are also located the blood vessels that serve part of the head of the femur. If the hip is dislocated, these blood vessels may be torn, and the bone will have no blood supply. This can lead to death of the bone in part of the head of the femur, which then requires major surgery. This is part of the reason why a hip dislocation is a very big deal; however, you're quite unlikely to dislocate your hip during yoga class.

The Labrum

Much like in the shoulder, the hip socket is deepened by a rim of cartilage known as the labrum. This structure further increases the contact of the femur with the acetabulum, spreads out the forces within the joint, and distributes synovial fluid more evenly. You can see it in the illustration below as a circular rim around the outer part of the acetabulum.

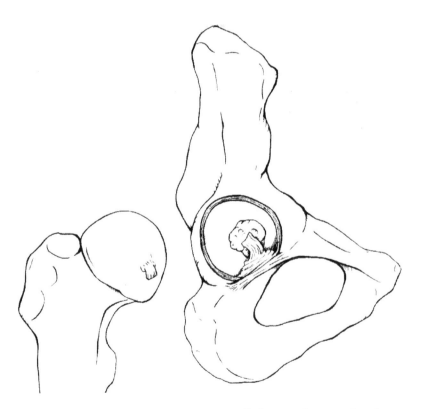

the femur and the acetabulum, pulled apart from each other

Because the femur and the acetabulum have so much surface area in direct contact, any actions that bring the femur to the edges of its range of motion can begin to pinch the labrum in between the head of the femur and the acetabulum itself. This is known as femoroacetabular impingement, or FAI. It wears away the cartilage of the femur and the acetabulum, and can lead to tears of the labrum. It occurs when the hip is taken to the edge of its range of motion and then force continues to be applied.

An acute tear of the labrum can occur when the femur is dislocated from its position in the acetabulum. As previously mentioned, this type of dislocation is a very big deal, but is uncommon. Similar to in the shoulder, a dislocation will damage the labrum, leaving the joint permanently more likely to dislocate again in the same direction.

More commonly, a chronic tear of the labrum occurs. This is a common injury in dancers and gymnasts; the cultures of these sports encourage forcing the hips into extreme positions (such as transversal splits) that most hips simply cannot perform safely. As a result, many dancers and gymnasts end their careers in their early 30s. A torn hip labrum is extremely painful, and the healing takes a long time and is usually incomplete, since the labrum is made of cartilage.

A yoga practitioner can also tear the labrum by attempting to force the hip into extreme positions. It's common for people to see photos of others in beautiful yoga poses, and to attempt to copy those shapes with their own bodies. While some hips will be able to handle this type of activity, for others, it will be hugely problematic, and could potentially cause damage.

Ligaments

The hip joint has a strong and thick joint capsule, and is supported by some of the strongest ligaments in the body. Strong connective tissue wraps the whole joint, holding the head of the femur into the acetabulum. Studies have indicated that the iliofemoral ligament, which is one of these ligaments, is the strongest ligament in the body.

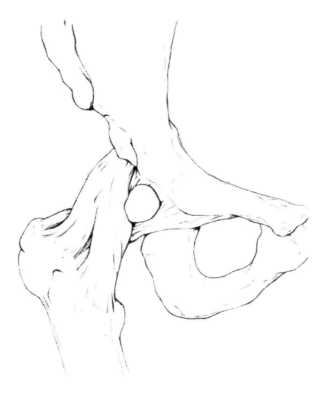

hip ligaments

In the illustration above, you can see many of these ligaments connecting to the pelvis and the femur. The small circle visible outside of the ligaments is a bursa.

Range of Motion

The hip joint can perform six basic movements (three pairs of movements). These are similar to the movements that are possible at the glenohumeral joint of the shoulder, although how large the movements can be is quite different in the hips.

Flexion of the hip draws the thigh toward the front of the torso (or the torso toward the thigh). Extension brings the leg behind the body.

When the hip abducts, the leg moves out to the side, away from the body. When it adducts, the leg moves toward and even across the midline of the body.

External rotation of the hip brings an imaginary line on the front of the thigh toward the outside of the body. This would direct the toes outward (although rotation at the knee can also affect the direction of the toes; see Chapter 12 for more on this). When the hip internally rotates, that line is turned toward the midline of the body, which tends to point the toes inward.

Now let's explore some of the issues involved with these movements, and how to ensure that you stay safe while you perform them.

Flexion

When you perform a forward bend, such as a seated forward bend (paschimottanasana), you're flexing your hips. At some point, you'll hit the end of your range of motion. Almost everyone believes that their hamstrings are what's limiting them. "Once I loosen my hamstrings," they believe, "I'll be able to lay my chest down on my thighs in the perfect forward bend."

There are undoubtedly people whose hamstrings are the major limitation on their range for hip flexion. Almost everyone is in this category when they begin their yoga practice. However, there are others, particularly those who have been practicing yoga for quite some time, who are limited not by tension in their hamstrings, but by the range of motion for flexion in their hips.

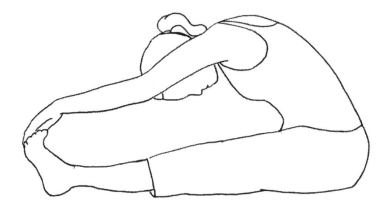

paschimottanasana

The average range of motion for flexion of the hip is about 120° to 140°. That's not quite 180°, which is what many yoga practitioners are striving for when they try to lay the chest down on the thighs. By adding flexion of the spine, the chest may still hit the thighs for some people; however, to get there with a completely flat spine is unlikely to be a healthy goal, and for many people, trying to force the chest to touch the thighs will cause damage in the hip.

When you go into a forward bend, feel your hip joint. Remember that it's in the groin region, near the front of your body. If you get pinching or squeezing there as you come forward, then you've hit the end of your range of motion for flexion. Attempting to force yourself to flex farther can lead to FAI (femoroacetabular impingement; i.e., bone touching bone), damaging the cartilage and potentially causing joint problems like osteoarthritis. If your hip joint is sore when you come out of the pose, then you're most likely damaging it; however, even if it's not sore, you could be causing damage, because cartilage doesn't always feel pain. Feel for compression, and back out of the pose slightly when you feel it.

Extension

The hip's range of motion for extension is, on average, very small. A normal range of extension is about 10 to 15°. The upper end of normal could be up to 40° – far less than the 90° that would be required to do the longitudinal splits (front-to-back splits, also known in yoga as hanumanasana) with the hips perfectly squared.

If you take a close look at most people doing longitudinal splits, you'll notice something: the yoga practitioner's pelvis is anteverted. (Recall from Chapter 7 that an anteverted pelvis is tipped forward.) This is what makes the splits possible. Rather than 90° of flexion and 90° of extension, as would be required if the pelvis were in neutral rotation, this pelvic anteversion allows the front hip to be more flexed and the back hip less extended. Since 90° of hip extension is, for most people, far more than is possible (even if their muscles are all extremely flexible, the bones and connective tissue will cause a limit), while 140° of flexion is within the range of possibility for most people, it's necessary to shift the pose to make it more about hip flexion than about hip extension.

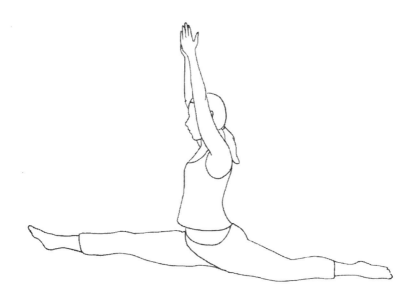

longitudinal splits

When the hip goes into deep extension, the front of the hip is pushed forward out of the socket. The contact between the femur and the acetabulum is decreased. This gives the practitioner an uncomfortable feeling of instability; it's not pain, exactly, but it's definitely not pleasant. If extension continues, damage to the labrum and even dislocation of the hip joint can result.

If you decide to start working toward longitudinal splits, be very aware of both hips, especially the back hip. Don't force it into deep extension. You may need to allow your pelvis to tip forward to decrease the extension of the back hip, but as you do this, beware of causing excessive flexion in the front hip.

If you get to a point where both hips feel compression, then you're at the end of your range of motion for the splits. If it turns out that your hips have 125° of safe flexion and 15° of safe extension, then your legs are never safely going to be 180° apart. You can be an excellent yoga practitioner who chooses not to do the splits; if it's not right for your body, then the best course of action is to let it go, rather than to try to force the pose and potentially damage your hips. You don't win yoga class by doing the splits perfectly (despite what many images in the media would like you to believe).

Extension comes up in other poses, too. For instance, the back hip in warrior 1 is in extension. Again, the pelvis is usually tipped forward to accommodate the limited extension of the back hip; with the torso fully upright, this can sometimes cause a significant extension (arch) in the low back.

Some yoga teachers insist that the pelvis is not supposed to be anteverted in this pose. However, forcing the pelvis to be upright instead of allowing it to tip forward could force the back hip into too much extension. This is an example of a traditional alignment cue that is not only not helpful from a safety point of view, but could actually be harmful. Allowing the pelvis to tip forward is safer for the hip, although it could cause pain in the low back due to hyperextension in some people.

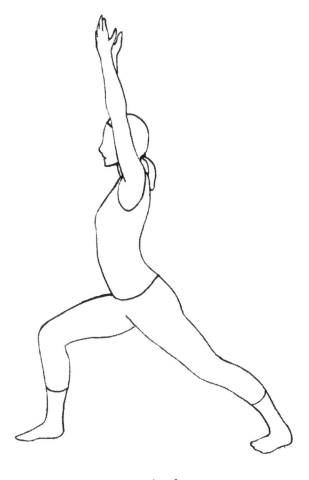

warrior 1

If the extension in the low back in warrior 1 is too much, you may be able to fix it by taking a smaller step backward as you come into the pose. You could also bring the back heel up into the variation often known as crescent lunge, and then bend the knee as much as necessary to reduce the extension in the back hip. (Bending the knee with the back heel down, as in warrior 1, puts too much torque on the knee.) Another option is to lean the torso forward on an angle, which reduces the extension in the back hip as well as the extension in the lumbar spine.

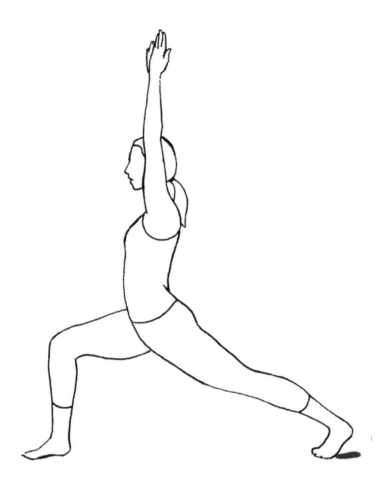

crescent lunge

If the low back doesn't hurt in warrior 1, then there's no reason that you shouldn't allow the pelvis to antevert. Given that the forward tilt of the pelvis protects the back hip from excessive extension, I believe it's best to allow it, despite its being against the traditional rules. I have yet to hear a convincing argument against this idea, beyond aesthetics.

Abduction

Abduction (bringing the leg out to the side away from the body) is normally limited to about 45°; that equates to a 90° angle between the legs when both hips are abducted. While going somewhat further than this is not uncommon, being able to do transversal splits (legs straight out to the sides) without damage to the hips is quite uncommon. There are very few hips that can tolerate 90° of abduction (per hip).

The range of abduction is generally limited by contact of the femoral neck with the pelvis. This will feel like a crowding or squeezing in the area of the hip joint, possibly a bit to the side of where you feel compression in deep hip flexion. As usual with compression, when you feel this sensation, it's the end of your safe range of motion; while you can probably squeeze out a little bit more range if you force your body deeper into the pose, doing this could irreparably damage your hips.

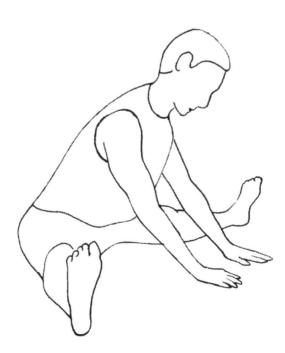

seated angle (upavista konasana)

However, many people do have tight adductor muscles (on the inner part of the thigh) and medial hamstrings (on back of the thigh, toward the inside), which can also limit the range of abduction. If you feel a stretch in your inner thigh as you abduct your hips, this is muscular tension, and it can safely be released and your range likely expanded. Remember to keep the sensation in the belly of the muscle, rather than near the joints, as you gently allow the fascia and muscle tissue to open while protecting the tendons and ligaments.

If you're feeling tension limiting the pose, you may be able to get a sense of which muscles are tight with a very simple exercise. Take seated angle pose (upavista konasana), and then bound angle pose (baddha konasana).

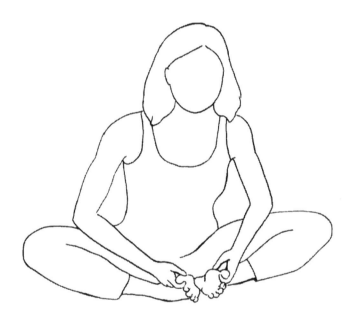

bound angle (baddha konasana)

If both poses are tight, and you feel tension in the inner thigh as you do them both, then it's likely to be your adductors that have tightness. These muscles cross only the hip, and aren't affected by bending the knee.

However, if bound angle is significantly more open than seated angle, and it's muscle tension that limits you, then it's likely that your medial hamstrings that are the culprits. If you push yourself too far into seated angle pose, you'll start to feel the stretch behind your knee toward the inside, and near your sit bone; these are the two attachments of the medial hamstring tendons. Back out from the pose until you feel the stretch in the belly of the muscle, and allow it to open gently.

There's more than just muscle tension going on here, however. In bound angle, the hips are held in external rotation; in seated angle, they're generally in neutral rotation. There's a greater range of abduction while in external rotation. For nearly everyone, after the muscle tension has been worked out and the limitations are within the joint itself, baddha konasana will be a more open pose than upavista konasana. If this is the case for you, both poses will be limited by compression in the hip joints rather than tension in the thighs.

External and Internal Rotation

If you swivel your legs from side to side, you're exploring external and internal rotation of the hips. Those with longer, thinner femoral necks generally have a greater range of motion for rotation in both directions. On average, women have a greater range for hip rotation than do men, although there's plenty of individual variation.

Remember that, as with all hip movements, there's an endpoint to the safe range of motion for rotation that's determined by the shape of the bones. To protect your labrum from impingement between the femur and the acetabulum, it's important to honor this limit.

One common cue in pigeon pose is to start working the lower leg to be parallel to the top of the mat (like the top illustration on the next page). Most people do the pose most comfortably with the front heel tucked in toward the opposite hip (like the bottom illustration on the next page), which requires a smaller degree of external rotation.

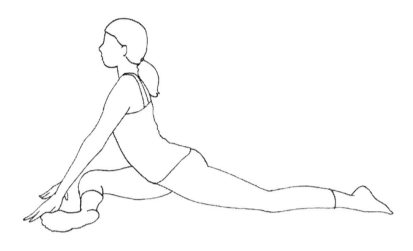

pigeon, with lower leg parallel to top of mat

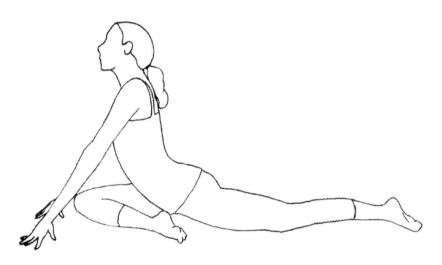

pigeon, with lower leg tucked in

When they're told that the goal is to get the shin parallel to the front of the mat, they begin to force that to happen. Many yoga students grab their foot with their hand and start pulling it toward the front of the mat.

Despite the pinch or even the pain they feel in the hip joint as they pull the leg forward in this way, many yoga practitioners stay in the pose, "breathing into the discomfort," and find that their hips are sore when they come out. (There's also a potentially deleterious effect on the knee, as we'll explore in the next chapter. Knee pain in pigeon is actually rather common, in my experience, and most people don't know why it happens.)

Similarly, most hips don't have enough external rotation to do lotus pose. As we'll see, when people try to force it, the knees take the brunt of this action. While lotus can be a problem for the hips, it's actually even more of a problem for the knees, so I'm saving this discussion for the next chapter.

How the Hips Affect the SI Joints

When the innominate bones move forward, coming closer together at the pubic symphysis, they spread apart slightly at the back, and the SI joints experience a stretch ("distraction"). Imagine the two hip crests winging forward, closing the front of the pelvis and opening the back of it. This is associated with internally rotating the hips.

When the innominate bones move back, they squish the SI joints ("compression"). Imagine the hip crests winging outward, opening somewhat like a book, with the back of the pelvis closing and the front opening. This is associated with externally rotating the hips.

The sacrum is a symmetrical structure. It doesn't tend to tolerate too much asymmetrical movement around it. When the pelvis is moved asymmetrically, then there can be compression (squeezing) at one SI joint and distraction (spreading apart) at the other one. While either of the joints could feel this sensation, it's usually the compressed joint that ends up hurting. Of course, some asymmetry is not a problem; there's an asymmetry created in the pelvis with every step you take. However, when asymmetry is forced too deep, or when movements are chronically asymmetrical in the same direction, it can become a problem.

How can you use this knowledge to protect the SI joints? Consider the rotation of both hips as an important part of creating space in your low back. For healthy SI joints, internal rotation of the hips will create more space than external rotation, and asymmetry can be problematic.

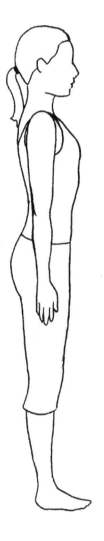

mountain pose

The gluteus maximus, the large muscle of the buttocks, is one of the main muscles that causes hip extension (bringing the leg behind the body). It's also a strong external rotator of the hip. Many people walk with their toes turned slightly out; the glutes are working to extend the hips during walking, and they will also tend to produce external rotation unless this is consciously opposed by other muscles. (Now that you're looking for it, you'll probably start to notice this phenomenon all the time.)

When you stand in tadasana (mountain pose), you may notice a tendency for your hips to be externally rotated, because of the external rotation produced by the glutes. Drawing them in, so your toes point straight forward, helps to create space in the lower back. Imagine that you have a block between your thighs (or, even better, actually put one there), and send the block behind you; that internally rotates your thighs slightly, creating additional space for the SI joints.

When you go into any pose that includes hip extension, the glutes will tend to bring the hips into external rotation. For instance, as you press up into bridge pose, the tendency is to use the glutes, because they're powerful hip extensors. However, using the glutes also tends to bring the hips into external rotation (you'll notice that the knees spread apart as this happens). The problem with that is that both SI joints will be compressed by the external rotation of the hips, and when you're trying to backbend, compression in the low back isn't really what you're aiming for. Bringing the knees closer together, so the hips are in neutral rotation, will help to create more space in the low back.

Strongly asymmetrical poses, like the twisting pose known as "half lord of the fishes pose" or ardha matsyendrasana, can cause one SI joint to be compressed while the other is distracted (spread apart). Notice in the illustration that the bottom leg is externally rotated, compressing the SI joint, while the top leg is internally rotated. Additionally, when you twist toward the internally rotated side, the SI joint will be compressed even more on the opposite (bottom leg) side. In yoga therapy, twists like this are used for SI joint problems; the practitioner twists only toward the painful side, avoiding the opposite side.

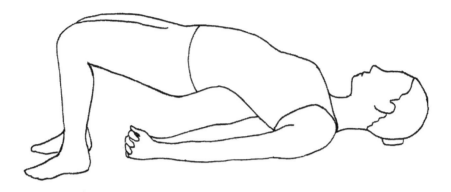

bridge pose

It's not just in yoga that awareness of your SI joints is useful. I've had quite a few yoga students mention to me that they wake up with SI joint pain every morning. Commonly, their sleep position is on one side, with one leg straight, and the other leg bent. When someone sleeps in this position, it's common to roll slightly onto the belly, so that the top leg is in external rotation. This is an asymmetrical position, and can cause compression of the SI joint on the top leg side. The risk that the SI joint will feel discomfort is magnified if the sleeper has a preferred side to sleep on, causing the same SI joint to be routinely compressed.

If you prefer side sleeping, it's best to keep both knees bent rather than just one, to protect the SI joint. Additionally, you should aim to keep both hips in neutral rotation. To do that, you need to have a pillow between both the knees and the ankles. When a pillow is placed just between the knees (as is common), then the top hip is pushed into external rotation, compressing the top SI joint. Putting the pillow between both the knees and the ankles keeps the hips aligned. (That means you can't hug the pillow, unfortunately. You can always have a second smaller pillow for hugging if you'd like.)

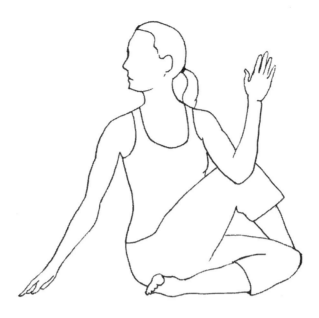

ardha matsyendrasana

How To Protect Your Hips

- Avoid forcing the hip into any range of motion that causes pain, squeezing, pinching, or a feeling of crowding in the joint, to protect the labrum and articular cartilage.
- If you choose to perform the splits (hanumanasana), allow the pelvis to antevert, to avoid excessive extension of the back hip. This protects both ligaments and cartilage. Similarly, allow pelvic anteversion in warrior 1 and other hip extension poses.
- Honor the limits of external and internal rotation of your hip. Don't attempt to force excessive rotations, to protect the cartilage of the hip.

The hip and the knee affect each other in significant ways. I've already mentioned a few poses in which limitations at the hip can cause damage at the knee. In the next chapter, we'll explore why this happens, and what you can do to protect your knees. If you've ever had knee pain in lotus or pigeon, the next chapter will help you.

CHAPTER 12:
THE KNEES

The knee is the most commonly injured joint in the limbs. While the hip is more stable than the shoulder, reflecting its need to bear the body weight, the knee is actually one of the least stable joints in the body. Estimates vary, but some official estimates suggest that up to ¼ of the population is experiencing knee pain at any given time.

Most of this knee pain is due to osteoarthritis, the wear and tear damage from our daily activities. Given the knee's lack of stability, everyday activities can damage it. Yoga definitely has the potential to cause or worsen knee damage.

Yet, by strengthening the muscles that protect the knee in a balanced way, yoga also has the potential to prevent knee damage. How can you do it the right way? Let's start with a quick look inside the knee.

The Bones

The knee is made up of three bones: the femur (thighbone), the tibia (shinbone), and the patella (kneecap).

At its proximal (top) end, the head of the femur fits into the acetabulum at the hip joint. At its distal (bottom) end, the femur has two rounded surfaces, called condyles, with a groove between them. These fit into two cups on the tibia, which are also called condyles (probably to make things as confusing as possible, which was the apparent goal of the early anatomists who named these structures).

In each cup is a cartilage structure called a meniscus (plural: menisci). These structures are somewhat similar to the labrum of the shoulder or hip; they increase the contact between the bones and spread out the forces of the joint. Each meniscus is shaped like a C, with the round part of the C on the outside of the knee. Only the ends of the C are attached; the rest of the meniscus can and does move when the knee moves. Some studies of yoga practitioners indicate that the meniscus is one of the bodily structures that's most commonly injured during yoga practice.

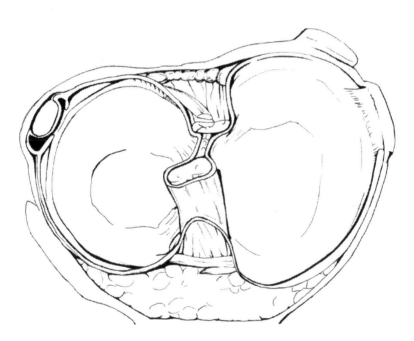

the two menisci, inside the knee

The knee is stabilized by a few ligaments, some of which are familiar to most people. There's a high likelihood that someone you know has torn their ACL at some point; the ACL is one of four main ligaments in the knee. The two collateral ligaments (the MCL and LCL) run along the sides of the knee, and the two cruciate ligaments (the ACL and PCL) cross through the knee's center from front to back.

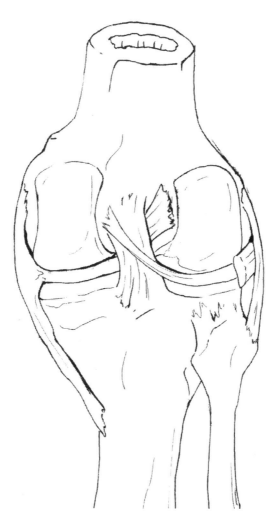

knee with ligaments; femur above, tibia below

In the illustration above, you can see the femur on the top and the tibia below; the cruciate ligaments are the X in the center, and the collateral ligaments are on the sides. (You can also see the fibula at the lower right of the illustration. This is a bone of the lower leg, but isn't involved in the knee joint; we'll discuss it in the next chapter.) Together, these structures provide some stability for the joint. However, given the large forces that the knee joint must be capable of bearing, this isn't a whole lot of connective tissue.

Range of Motion

Most people think of the knee as a hinge joint, which can flex (bend) and extend (straighten). While the knee does have a hinge action, it's more complicated than that. The knee is a compound joint, rather than a pure hinge (like the elbow). Along with the hinge movement, the femoral condyles glide on the tibia as the knee moves.

The knee does flex and extend, and when it's in flexion, it has some ability to rotate as well. The lower leg can internally or externally rotate relative to the upper leg. When the knee is in extension, it's prevented from rotating by the tautness of the ligaments. Knowledge of this ability of the knee to rotate is one of the main keys to protecting it.

Knee Rotation

Consider the two poses on the following two pages. One is lotus pose (padmasana), and the other is hero's pose (virasana). Notice how, in lotus, the lower leg is folded towards the inside of the upper leg, while in virasana, the lower leg is outside of the upper leg. In other words, the knee is in internal rotation in one pose, and external rotation in the other. (There's also a difference in the hip rotation in these poses, but we're focusing on the knees here.)

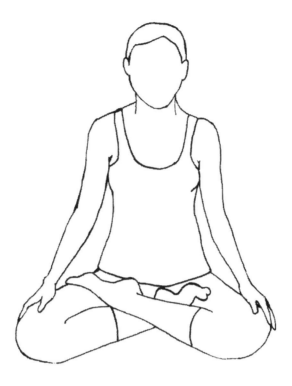

lotus pose

Rotation of the knees is normal, and is necessary during walking, because the lateral (outer) condyles are larger than the medial (inner) condyles, and therefore need to move farther. (You can see this in the earlier illustration of the two menisci; the lateral one, pictured on the right, is larger than the medial one, pictured on the left.) However, while rotation is normal, excessive rotation puts pressure on the structures of the knee and can damage them. The cartilage can be worn away, or the meniscus can be damaged.

If you're like many yoga students, you may have seen the photos of these poses and thought, "Both of those poses make my knees hurt." Why?

Take a look at the hips in lotus; the pose requires a lot of external rotation there. When the hips don't quite have enough external rotation to come into lotus, but the practitioner is determined to sit in the pose anyway, he or she can force it through extra rotation of the knees. People often grab each foot and yank it up into the opposite hip crease, however much force this takes. Remember, some knee rotation is fine, but too much knee rotation causes pain. So when the lack of hip rotation is compensated for by excessive knee rotation, knee pain is the result.

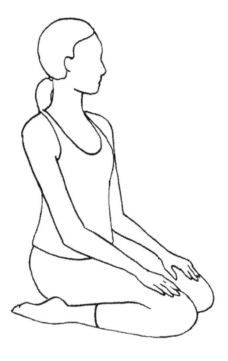

hero's pose (virasana)

This is why I believe that lotus is one of the most dangerous yoga positions. Many people are determined to sit in lotus, because they believe that yogis are supposed to sit that way. And, unfortunately, some of the "classic" teachings tell us that, if your knees hurt in lotus, you should just keep sitting in the pose anyway. The pain will go away eventually.

When yoga practitioners get knee osteoarthritis, I don't believe that they're more enlightened as a result.

If lotus hurts your knees, sitting in lotus is really not worth it. There's nothing magical about lotus pose. Instead, just take a regular cross-legged seat that feels good on your knees. Notice how, in a cross-legged seat, the knees (and hips) are far less rotated. This is also a classic meditation pose, with a fancy Sanskrit name (sukhasana), and is completely valid as a way to sit in meditation.

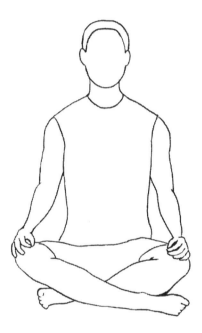

sukhasana

Remember that how far the hips can externally rotate is constrained by the shape of the bones. If you can't sit in lotus without knee pain, then maybe it's because of muscle tightness, and you'll get flexible enough to do it eventually. However, even after releasing any tension in their leg and hip muscles, many people still can't sit in lotus without knee issues. In modern Western societies, where hips are formed while sitting in chairs, this is particularly common.

Because lotus is problematic for most people's bodies, I don't encourage people to take this pose in my classes. Even for those with a big range of external rotation, getting the tops of the feet up into the hip creases often causes a significant knee rotation. And unless you're going to be throwing your lotused legs around (like in a handstand), there's really no advantage to doing this. So why put the extra wear and tear on your knees?

Hero's pose, or virasana, requires a big hip rotation the opposite way (an internal rotation). Again, whether or not your hips can do this is related to the shape of your bones, and there's really nothing "more advanced" about being able to get a larger range of internal rotation of the hips.

I hear many people tell me that virasana hurts their knees. It could be related to the knee flexion; not all knees flex far enough to sit back on your heels. Often, though, knee pain in virasana is related to excessive knee rotation, which is related to trying to do the pose with insufficient internal rotation at the hip – very similar to what happens in lotus with insufficient external rotation.

If virasana hurts your knees, please don't just push through this pain! The fix is simple: sit on something – a block, a bolster, whatever you have around. Put it between your heels, tuck your heels all the way next to it, and sit on it. This reduces the amount of internal rotation required at the hip, so that the knees don't have to rotate to make the pose happen. You can still get plenty "advanced" with the pose; you can even lean your torso all the way back to get that big hip flexor stretch, if it feels like a good idea. (Don't feel like you "must" or even "should" lean all the way back, however.)

Once you're aware of the knee rotation issue, you'll start noticing it in other poses, too. Pigeon is another one where people try to "fake" a bigger hip rotation with extra knee rotation. If pigeon hurts your forward knee, then that's what's happening. When people try to get the lower leg parallel to the front of the mat, and grab the foot to crank it up there, the knee experiences way too much rotation in most people and will get sore.

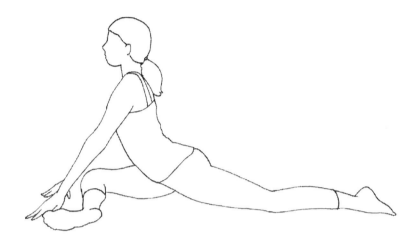

pigeon, with lower leg parallel to top of mat

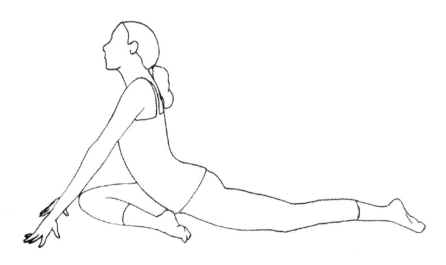

pigeon, with lower leg tucked in

To prevent this, tuck your front heel in more toward your body, which reduces both the hip and knee rotation and prevents damage to the knee. The goal is to find a variation of pigeon that doesn't hurt your knee at all. That might look like the bottom illustration below, or it might be somewhere in between the two options shown; see what works in your body.

Knee rotation also comes up in standing poses. Think about your back heel in warrior 1. With the heel down, there's a hip rotation. The cue is often then given to square the hips toward the front of the mat. With the foot fixed and the femur moving, but potentially not mobile enough to achieve adequate hip rotation, the knee may be subjected to excessive rotation.

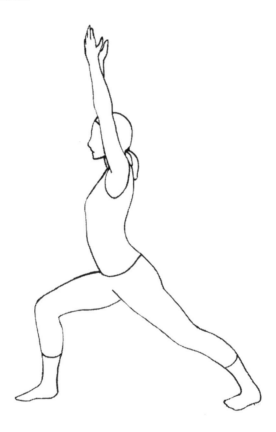

warrior 1

Because of this issue, I recommend against squaring the hips to the front of the mat in warrior 1. That's an old cue, and the only reason I can see to do it is that it's prettier. Instead, allow the hips to point toward the front corner of the mat, on the side with the leg back (i.e., in warrior 1 with the right leg forward and the left leg back, the hips will point a little to the left), which is the natural direction for them anyway. This is preferable, because it creates less torque on the knee.

Knee rotation comes up off the mat, too. For example, if your knees hurt after you run, this could be the reason; paying attention to how your feet are oriented when they land is helpful.

Protecting the Patella

The patella, or kneecap, is interesting in that it's a sesamoid bone. That means it's located within a tendon. Not attached to a tendon; *inside* of one. There are few bones like this in the body, and no other one nearly as big as the patella. (Side note: Babies don't have kneecaps! There's a little cartilage, but no bone there. The patella forms months later, in response to forces placed on the tendon. This lack of kneecaps is part of why baby knees look so pudgy and cute.)

The tendon the patella is within is the quadriceps tendon. You can find this tendon easily if you feel just below your kneecap; that bump on the front of your tibia near the top is where the tendon inserts. The top of the patella is shaped like a dome, and can be easily felt below the skin. The bottom of the patella is shaped like a wedge, which glides in the groove between the condyles of the femur.

It's very important that the patella stays within its groove. If it deviates to one side or the other, the cartilage on the underside of the patella gets damaged. You may have heard someone say that it hurts under his or her kneecap. That's the result of chronic knee deviation.

Fortunately, the way to keep the patella safe in yoga is fairly simple and is commonly cued in yoga classes. Whenever bending the knee with weight on it, keep the knee facing directly forward (over the middle of the foot, which is approximately the second toe). If the knee moves toward the inside or outside of the foot, the patella will be pressed against one side of its groove, and may experience damage. This cue applies to warrior poses, chair pose, and many others. It also applies to walking and running, and also to all of your other non-yoga activities.

Quadriceps is Latin for four heads. While the four parts of the quadriceps come together at the knee to form one tendon, they're separate muscles above that point. There's one on each side of the leg, one in the center, and another longer one in the center that reaches up over the hip.

For the patella to track healthfully in its groove, the four muscles need to pull on it in a balanced way. In particular, the two muscles on the sides need to pull equally. If one of them is stronger than the other, the patella will be pulled to one side every time the knee extends.

While significant imbalances in the strength of the quadriceps muscles are best addressed by physical therapy, you can consciously try to bring balance into this system by thinking about activating your whole thigh, not just a part of it, when you use your quadriceps. Place your hand gently over the front of your thigh as you straighten your knee, and feel the various muscles activating.

The "Knee Above Ankle" Cue

The other common knee cue you'll hear in yoga classes is "keep your knee above your ankle" during lunge poses (such as warriors). Yoga teachers believe that it's important to keep the knee directly above the ankle, rather than in front of it. This idea is controversial in the fitness world.

The origin of this cue lies in biomechanical studies from decades ago. Some research suggested that letting the knee come forward of the ankle would put excessive force on the knee joint, possibly leading to knee damage. However, later research suggested that, while the knee forward of the ankle may put extra force on the knee, keeping the knee directly above the ankle actually leads to extra force on the hip, meaning that neither one is necessarily better.

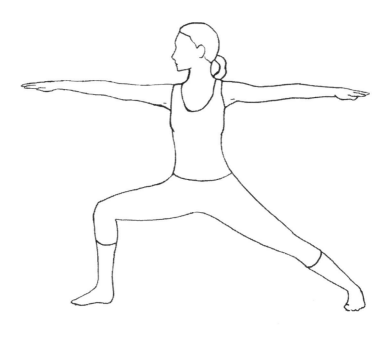

warrior 2

Some leading physical therapists have stated that having the knee forward of the ankle is not a problem, as long as there's enough strength to support the body weight, and the person is not leaning the weight excessively forward into that bent knee. Of course, when teaching a group yoga class, you can't be sure that people have the strength to support themselves and won't lean forward over the bent knee. Additionally, a knee forward of the ankle may be less stable and more likely to move to one side, which would not be good.

When I teach, I don't think of this as the most important aspect of lunge poses like warriors. However, I do find that keeping the knee directly above the ankle feels "stronger" and leads to more muscular engagement for most people than does letting it drift in front. For myself, I feel more stable and grounded in the pose when the knee is directly above the ankle. I will mention keeping the knee above the ankle and will demonstrate it that way, but am not terribly concerned if some people's knees come somewhat forward of their ankles. In some poses, such as chair pose, it's essentially impossible to keep the knee from coming forward of the ankle, and I see no reason to be concerned about that.

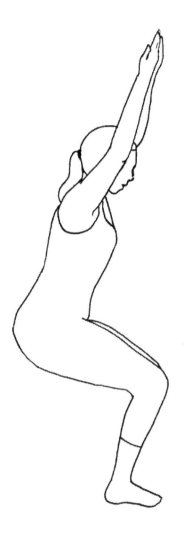

chair pose

Sideways Pressure on the Knee

Although it does rotate, the knee doesn't bend sideways. Because of this, pressure on the knee from the side (either side) causes forces within the knee that can damage the cartilage or the menisci.

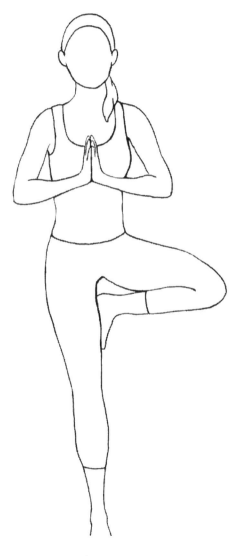

tree pose

This comes up mainly in tree pose, in which it's extremely important that the lifted foot is placed on the thigh or the calf, rather than on the knee itself. Make sure that the lifted foot feels like it's pressing into a bone and not a joint. If your toes graze your knee, that's fine, as long as the pressure is kept off.

"Hyperextension"

As discussed in the elbow chapter, hyperextension is one of the most misunderstood concepts in modern yoga practice. With the knee, as with the elbow, recurvation (a knee that goes beyond 180° when extended) is not necessarily a problem. It doesn't constitute "hyperextension," a term reserved for taking a joint into extension *beyond* its normal range of motion.

If your knees are recurved, your teacher may tell you to put a microbend in your knee. This means that you strengthen the muscles around the knee, bending it so slightly that it's hard to see that there's a bend at all. Whether the knee's normal range of motion is greater or less than 180°, microbending builds strength around the knee joint, helping to keep it protected from being forced past its normal range of motion in any direction. However, microbending will cause you to come out of poses earlier because of muscle fatigue. For more on this issue, see the discussion of elbow "hyperextension" in Chapter 9.

The Popliteal Vein

There is a reason not to keep the knees locked for a long period of time. The hollow behind the knee is called the popliteal fossa, and it contains the popliteal vein and the popliteal artery (among other structures).

When the knee is completely locked, the popliteal vein may be compressed. This doesn't happen in everyone; it depends on the individual anatomy. Some people can lock their knees for hours without compressing the popliteal vein, while others experience symptoms from even a few minutes of locking. (The artery will not usually be compressed, because arteries have thick muscular walls that resist compression, while veins have thin floppy walls.)

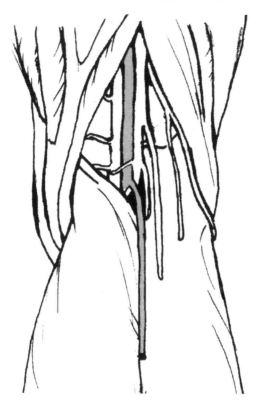

popliteal fossa (popliteal vein highlighted in gray)

If the popliteal vein is compressed, then blood becomes trapped in the lower legs, unable to get back to the heart because of the closed vein. Slowly, as more and more blood is trapped in the legs, less and less becomes available for important things – like maintaining consciousness. The person faints.

This kind of thing happens in the military, when soldiers stand at attention for hours at a time. It's pretty unlikely to happen in yoga, just because we don't usually stand still for that long. However, if you're standing in mountain pose (tadasana) with your knees locked, and if you stay there for several minutes (which may occur in some classes, if this pose is being used to teach mindfulness, or if it's a beginner's class in which mountain pose is explained in detail), then it's possible that you'll get dizzy. To avoid this, put a microbend in your knees.

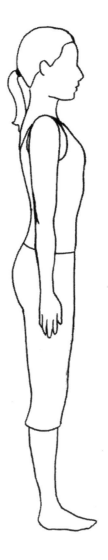

mountain pose

Hamstrings

If you feel the space behind your knee, you'll find a diamond shape, made from tendons above and below. The tendons coming down to cross your knee joint from above are the tendons of the hamstrings. (If you feel carefully, you'll find one on the outside and two on top of each other on the inside.)

The hamstrings cross two joints: the hip and the knee. They extend the hip (draw it backwards) and flex the knee (bend it). That means they're stretched when you flex the hip (bend forward from the hip) and extend the knee (straighten it).

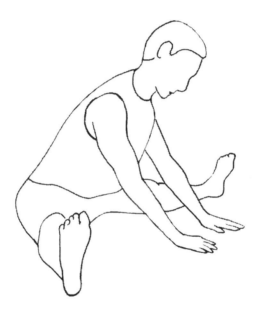

seated wide-legged forward bend (upavista konasana)

Many yoga poses stretch the hamstrings. When going into a forward bend with your knees straight, you may start to feel sensation in the hamstring tendons on either side of the knee. This is an unsafe sensation and needs to be addressed, to prevent these tendons from being permanently stretched out. I usually recommend bending the knee, although you could also unfold from the hips a little. Either way, it's important to relieve the stretch on the hamstrings to protect the tendons.

In upavista konasana (seated wide-legged forward bend), the hamstrings are stretched, particularly the ones on the inner side of the thigh. I find that it's common for people to report a deep stretch behind the inner part of the knee, resulting from the tendon being pulled on as the muscle is taken into a very deep stretch. You should address this by backing out of the pose a little to reduce the stretch.

How To Protect Your Knees

- Watch out for excessive knee rotation, to protect the menisci and the cartilage of the knee joint.
- Don't use rotation of the knee to compensate for a smaller range of motion in the hip.
- Ensure that the knee bends straight forward instead of drifting inward or outward, to protect the cartilage of the patella.
- Don't put pressure on the knee from the side, such as in tree pose, to protect the articular cartilage of the knee.
- Locking the knee is okay, even if your knee naturally goes beyond 180°; just don't stay there too long.
- Pain or a deep stretch sensation in the hamstring tendons behind the knee is an unsafe sensation. Bend the knees or come out of the forward bend slightly until you feel the sensation in the belly of the muscle and not in the tendons.
- If your knee hurts, take the warning seriously and come out of or modify the pose.

To complete our tour of the leg, the next chapter will explore the ankles and feet. If you've been told that you have "flat feet," or have experienced ankle pain in poses like hero's pose (virasana), this chapter will help you learn more about these issues and what you can do about them.

CHAPTER 13:
THE ANKLES AND FEET

Our feet are the platforms on which we stand, and yet our awareness of them is often rudimentary. Problems in the foot and ankle often lead to problems further up in the knee and hip, as the posture is adjusted to compensate. Knowledge of our foundations is key to keeping our bodies safe during yoga practice.

Bones

As we saw in the last chapter, there are two bones in the lower leg: the tibia and the fibula. Unlike the forearm, which has two bones that are relatively the same size, the lower leg has one large bone (the tibia) and one smaller bone (the fibula). In the illustration below, the fibula is the one on the left, toward the outside of the foot.

The tibia and the fibula each end in a bony bump called a malleolus, from the Latin for "hammer." (Remember the stylus process of the ulna and the stylus process of the radius? These are similar structures, but bigger.) Together, these two processes form a structure shaped somewhat like a wrench (not like a hammer, as their names might

191

suggest).

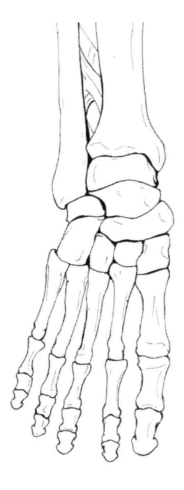

bones of the ankle and foot (tibia, fibula, tarsals, metatarsals, phalanges)

The tarsals are the ankle bones. The "wrench" formed by the tibia and fibula pinches the upper tarsal, which is called the talus (TALE-us). The talus rests on top of the bony calcaneus (cal-CANE-ee-us), or heel bone. There are five other tarsals, which are roughly similar in structure to the carpals of the wrist; they're small bones with gliding joints between them, bound together with lots of connective tissue.

From the tarsals, the metatarsals originate. These are the bones of the midfoot. They form the arch of the foot, which we'll discuss shortly. At the end of each metatarsal are several phalanges; there are three in each toe, except two in the big toe.

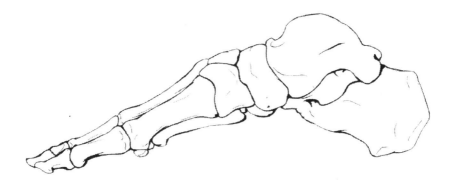

bones of the foot (tarsals, metatarsals, and phalanges)

In the illustration above, the calcaneus is the large bone on the right. You can see the talus above, and the other tarsals as you move toward the left, followed by the metatarslas and phalanges. You're looking at the big toe side of this foot.

Range of Motion

At the ankle joint, the foot can make two different movements that are both called flexion (just to make things less clear). When the top of the foot moves toward the lower leg, that's called dorsiflexion. When the sole of the foot moves downward (as in pointing your toe or wearing high heels), that's called plantar flexion. (In truth, plantar flexion is actually flexion, and dorsiflexion is extension. Think of the back of the hand coming toward the arm; that's wrist extension. The top of the foot coming toward the leg is ankle extension. However, most people think of that movement as "flexing the foot," so it gets called dorsiflexion instead of extension.)

The joint can also make two other movements. When the sole of the foot turns inward, that's called inversion, or sometimes supination. (This movement is structurally quite different from the forearm rotation that's also called supination, but it results in a position of the foot that's similar to that of the hand when the forearm is supinated.) When the sole of the foot moves outward, that's called eversion, or pronation. As we'll see, walking with the foot held in one of these positions can cause problems.

The toes have the same abilities as the fingers: they can flex and extend, and can abduct and adduct.

The Arch of the Foot

Together, the tarsals and metatarsals form the arch of the foot. Notice that your foot has an arch from front to back, and another arch from inner edge to outer edge.

The arch of the foot is malleable. Each time the foot hits the ground, the arch flattens slightly, and springs back up as the foot leaves the ground again. This is why stiff "arch support" in shoes is not a good idea; the arches actually need to be able to move, collapsing a bit with each step.

Those who are "flat-footed" often have an issue, not with the bones, but with the muscles and connective tissue that hold the arch of the foot in place. They may walk with their feet slightly everted (pronated), so the pressure of the step is landing more directly on the arch. Try walking with the majority of your weight on the outer edge of your foot, and then try walking with your feet slightly turned so that the weight falls more on the arch. You'll notice that your arches flatten as you put your weight on them with your foot slightly everted.

To protect the arches during yoga, it's best to keep this from happening. We want the foot to stay strong to keep its shape.

In warrior 1 or 2, a lack of attention to the back foot may well cause the weight to fall directly on the arch. That's why it's necessary to pay attention to pressing through the outer edge of that back foot. If you try this pressing and then try the pose without it, you may notice how much more supported your arch feels when you're pressing through the outer edge of your foot. This is a slight inversion of your ankle, which is necessary to bring the sole of your foot down (in neutral rotation, the side of your foot would be resting on the mat, which is both uncomfortable and not ideal for your bones).

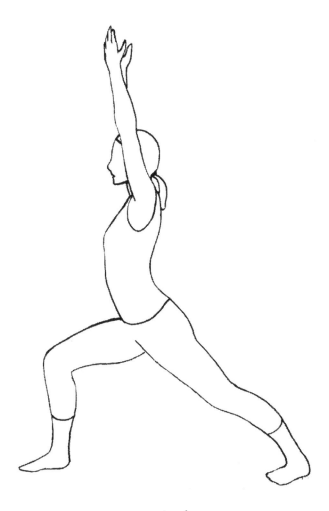

warrior 1

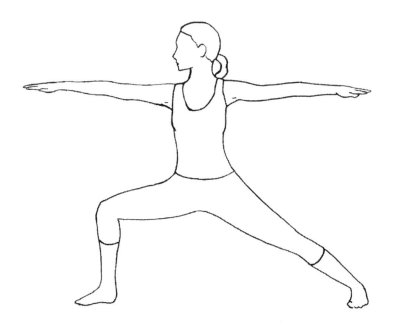

warrior 2

The "Four Corners" of the Feet

In mountain pose (tadasana), or other poses where you're standing on both feet, yoga teachers very commonly cue you to "bring your weight equally into all four corners of your feet." This cue is a good starting point to help those who tend to stand in pronation to begin correcting that problem.

However, I can't help pointing out that the foot doesn't really have four corners. A glance at the bottom of your foot will reveal three main places where your weight naturally falls: one over your calcaneus (your heel bone), and two on the ball of your foot (one on each side) over the ends of your metatarsals. So, if anything, it might make more sense to refer to the "three corners of the foot," as this may be easier for students to feel.

Consider the structure of those bones. The calcaneus is a huge and heavy bone. It's designed to transfer the weight of the body into the ground. The metatarsals are much smaller, and while they're capable of handling the entire body weight (as they do briefly, with each step), they're not designed to be the primary supporters of the body weight while standing. When you're well-aligned in standing poses like mountain, you'll feel your weight more toward your heels than toward the balls of your feet.

Walking with your weight primarily on the metatarsals, as people do when wearing shoes with high heels, can begin to cause problems with these bones. As the ends of the metatarsals take more force than they're able to handle, the bones begin to be damaged. Sometimes, bone spurs form; these are abnormal bone growths produced by a damaged bone. Podiatrists can remove them with surgery, but they may cause lots of pain in the meantime. It doesn't take a ton of heel height to cause this, either. Just a couple of inches of heel can cause this problem. Look at dress shoes for both men and women, and you'll see that this amount is common.

The Muscles of the Calf

In the calf, there are two large muscles that provide the power necessary to propel the body weight off the ground with each step. The outer one, called the gastrocnemius, has two tendons that cross the knee (it's also a knee flexor, meaning that it bends the knee, but it does so weakly). You may be able to feel these tendons behind the knee on the bottom. Its partner muscle, soleus, is located just underneath of it, and originates off the tibia itself (not crossing the knee).

Both of the muscles share a common tendon, called the Achilles (ah-KILL-eez) tendon. This is the thick tendon behind the ankle. (It's named after Achilles, the hero of Greek mythology, who was held by this tendon as an infant while his mother dipped him in the magical waters that made him impervious to harm; with the tendon undipped, he later died when an arrow pierced it.)

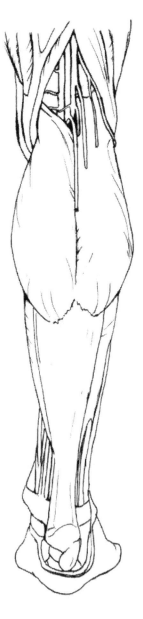

gastrocnemius muscle and Achilles tendon

Because the muscles attached to the Achilles tendon are plantar flexors (they point the toe), this tendon is under stretch when the ankle is dorsiflexed (the top of the foot is coming toward the lower leg). While active dorsiflexion of the foot in yoga is actually not very common, passive dorsiflexion occurs in poses like chair pose (utkatasana) and low squat (malasana).

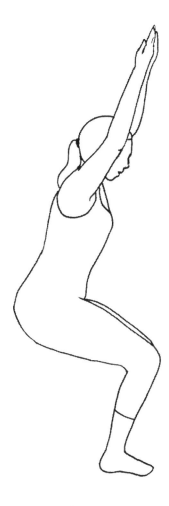

chair pose

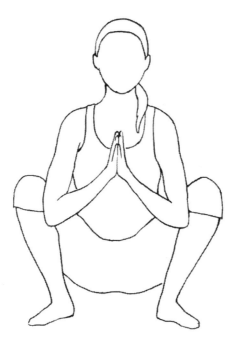

low squat (malasana)

Both of these poses have a tendency to cause pain in the ankle. People commonly feel it as pressure in the front of the ankle; that's compression, indicating the bony limit of dorsiflexion in that person's ankles. As with all compression, pushing into this sensation in hopes of changing the range of motion is neither safe nor effective.

Elevating the heels with a folded towel or folding up the mat can make these poses more comfortable as well as safer; simply allowing the ankles to float off the ground, with no attempt to force them to come down, is also an option. Not every body is skeletally structured in such a way that squatting with the pelvis very low and the heels down is possible; rather than coveting the shapes other people's bodies make in these poses, supporting your own body to protect its function long-term makes much more sense.

Sometimes, when the ankle reaches its limit for dorsiflexion, people feel a stretch in the Achilles tendon. Again, that's an unsafe sensation, as the tendon is being stretched. This indicates that there's an extreme stretch in the calf muscles (gastrocnemius and soleus). While stretching the tendon is unsafe, stretching the muscles and fascia is much safer. The range of motion will slowly expand over time, as the muscles of the calf become less tight.

The range of motion for plantar flexion also varies. While some people can lay the tops of their feet flat on the floor with no pain, others have a small space under the ankle. In hero's pose (virasana), it's rather common for people to have ankle pain. Sitting through the pain, forcing the ankle to plantar flex under the body weight, is not going to help. I've found that, for most people, simply rolling up two washcloths or small towels and placing one under each ankle gives the needed support, and prevents the ankle from being sore in this pose.

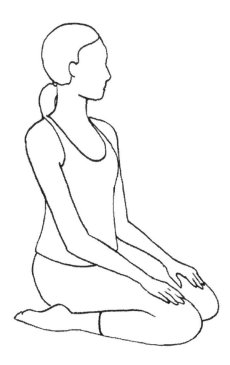

virasana

The Plantar Fascia

Along the bottom of each foot is a thick fascial covering known as the plantar fascia. This structure attaches at the heel and at the ball of the foot, covering the sole of the foot. This structure is stretched when the toes are extended. The plantar fascia has an unfortunate tendency to become inflamed at times. This condition is called plantar fasciitis (fash-ee-EYE-tis), and it causes uncomfortable tingling on the bottom of the foot.

Under the plantar fascia, there's a fat pad. This structure acts as a cushion for the bottom of the foot, which is subjected to body weight. Slowly, over time, the fat pad may be worn away, leaving the bottoms of the feet less protected. This causes the person to be vulnerable to plantar fasciitis, and to other causes of foot pain. (We all know of at least one older person whose feet hurt whenever he or she walks.)

This is my reason for being a little wary of the minimalist footwear that's currently popular, which puts only an extremely thin layer of shoe beneath the foot. There's no question that thick or stiff soles, particularly if they have "arch support," interfere with the function of the feet and can lead to problems. At the same time, however, having no cushion at all on the bottom of the foot could lead to the fat pad being worn down faster. Unfortunately, those wearing minimalist footwear as young adults won't know until much later whether this has happened. I don't know for certain that it will be a problem; however, I suspect that it might.

I believe that it's safer to use a shoe with a thin cushion on the bottom. This sole should be extremely flexible, so that it allows the foot to function well biomechanically, and should be relatively flat, so that it doesn't interfere with the changing shape of the arch during walking or running. There's currently a great deal of debate among podiatrists, biomechanical engineers, and other scientists about what type of shoe is ideal; if you're interested, you can find a lot more information about this topic in other resources.

The Muscles of the Foot

Much like in the hand, the foot is controlled mainly by muscles located outside of the foot itself. These muscles are in the lower leg, and they cross the ankle joint as well as the toe joints. The previously noted link between wrist position and finger position also applies to ankle position and toe position; in a plantar flexed ankle, the toes will not be able to achieve full flexion (curl inward). (See Chapter 10 for a discussion of the extrinsic muscles of the hand.)

There are a few muscles located in the foot itself, and again, they're similar to those in the hand. The muscles that spread the toes and bring them together are located in the foot, as well as groups of muscles that control the big toe and the little toe. (You may notice that you're able to spread your little toe apart from the others, but your middle three toes move as a group; if you're attentive, you will be able to feel the muscle in the outer edge of your foot working to cause that movement.)

The muscles of the foot and lower leg are vulnerable to cramping. Many people experience muscle cramps during their yoga practice or other exercise. One reason for these cramps is physical stress on the muscles; the muscles within the foot are working to maintain the arch whenever you're standing, and as you move through an exercise routine (which may put extra stress on them), you may cause small tears or other damage to these muscles. Damaged muscles tend to cramp, as they're unable to completely control the levels of ions within their cells. This type of cramps will be relieved by resting between exercise sessions, giving the muscles time to heal.

Cramps in the lower legs and feet are also common when the balance of minerals in the body is altered. When you're dehydrated, the minerals in your body are more concentrated. That makes muscle cramps more likely, and they'll tend to occur in the lower legs and feet. Drinking plenty of water before, during, and after your yoga practice can help to prevent these cramps.

Unfortunately, some yoga traditions fluid-restrict students, preventing them from getting the water they need during their practice. I do understand not wanting students to drink a huge amount of water, because it will expand their stomachs, which can be uncomfortable when turning upside down. Also, it tends to make people need to pee. However, fluid restriction while sweating has the potential to lead to a whole variety of problems, and foot cramps aren't even the worst of them.

I encourage students to drink water whenever they feel the need during classes, although I mention that chugging your whole water bottle is probably not going to feel so great. For myself, I drink a glass (or two) of water about half an hour before class. That gives the water time to be absorbed, and for me to pee before class starts. Then I only need small amounts during class, as I'm starting off hydrated. This staves off cramps, dizziness, and other dehydration-related issues, making my practice much more comfortable and safe.

The balance of the minerals sodium, potassium, calcium, and magnesium is crucial to the functioning of muscles; when this balance is disturbed, muscle cramps may result. While a full discussion of the possible mineral imbalances is beyond the scope of this book, you can ensure that you're getting enough of all of them by eating well (read: lots of veggies). If you get muscle cramps and they don't go away when you rest and hydrate, you should talk to your doctor about them, because they could be caused by a mineral imbalance or another medical condition.

How To Protect Your Ankles and Feet

- Avoid forcing the ankles to dorsiflex (top of the foot coming toward the lower leg) when the ankle joint is feeling compressed, to avoid damaging the cartilage. If desired, elevate the heels on a blanket or folded mat for support.
- Avoid forcing plantar flexion of the ankle under body weight, such as in virasana; support under the ankle with a rolled-up towel can help.

- Protect the arch of the foot by pressing into its outer edge, so you don't pronate (stand on the arch of the foot) in poses like the warrior poses. This protects the tissues of the arch.
- Stay hydrated during your practice, to prevent muscle cramps as well as dizziness and other problems.

We've now completed our tour of the body. You have a variety of tools to keep yourself safe during your yoga practice. I believe strongly in the benefits of yoga, and in its potential to be a lifelong practice that supports health and well-being. I'd like to leave you with a little yoga inspiration as you go forth into your practice.

CONCLUSION:
YOGA INSPIRATION

Throughout this book, I've offered you advice on how to practice yoga safely. My intention is not to convince you that yoga is unsafe and can hurt you, but rather to show you how you can adapt it to your own body and use it to benefit your health.

Yoga is for everybody. While most yoga teachers say this, and believe it, they don't necessarily know how to adapt the poses of yoga to work in every body. Bodies come in many shapes, and it's not just the soft tissues that are different.

Honor your bones and joints, and you will be able to practice for life. Keep your awareness of the principles described here, not only during your yoga practice, but throughout your daily activities and your other exercise. Increasing body awareness is a lifelong practice, and it won't be perfected overnight, but the path toward more body awareness holds great value. Yoga practice is an excellent tool for becoming aware of the ways in which we choose to hold and to move our bodies. When this awareness spreads off the yoga mat and into our lives, the benefits are enormous.

Strength allows you to keep your joints aligned for their health. Yoga poses that build strength are therefore protective for your joints, as long as you perform them with an eye toward safety. A side benefit of strength is that it allows you the freedom to do more with your life. When you're physically strong, you can do more activities, you can function more easily in your daily life, and you may even feel emotionally and mentally stronger, too.

Flexibility is also a key to health. While we're used to thinking of flexibility as a nice add-on to fitness, rather than an integral part of it, research is changing that view. Flexibility is correlated with health measures, such as better arterial health (translation: lower risk of stroke and heart attack) and better blood sugar control for diabetics. That doesn't mean extreme flexibility with no limits is the goal; pushing the limits of your flexibility too far can, as mentioned, damage your joints and leave your body unstable and prone to injury. As in all things, there's a balance. Finding your limits, and honoring them while creating optimal health, is the ideal.

I feel honored to be a teacher of yoga. This practice can be transformative, and every time I teach, a group of people trusts me to keep their bodies safe and to create a wellness-promoting experience for each of them. They open their hearts and their bodies. I'm incredibly honored by this trust.

I'm also honored to be a teacher of yoga teachers. When yoga teachers are given tools to keep people safe, the effect can ripple through many "generations" of yoga teachers; through the teachers I teach directly, and via their classes, to the yoga teachers that some of their students eventually become. So much of yoga is received wisdom handed down through the ages. Why not allow some of that received wisdom to be informed by modern scientific knowledge?

Above all, I find in the human body a source of endless wonder and fascination. The complexity of our bodies is astounding. Our ability to move through the world seamlessly, even without a detailed understanding of how everything works, is also astounding. It's a tragedy that so many people are taught anatomy in a dry, boring way that seems to bear no relationship to the bodies they actually live in. It puts them off wanting to explore deeper and learn more. I love to create a spark of interest in learning more about the body. Through each drop of knowledge we acquire, we become more empowered.

As you move through the world in your exquisitely complex body, may you live in ever-increasing wonder.

~~~~~~

I look forward to continuing the journey of exploration with you. You can check out my website, pattisheltonmd.com, where I have a blog, as well as information on my upcoming workshops, trainings, and retreats. If you have any questions, or would like to learn more about a topic, you can send me an email through the site. You can also sign up for my monthly email newsletter, in which I share my thoughts and insights as well as keep you up-to-date on my yoga-related activities.

Namaste, my friends, and I look forward to continuing to serve you. May you be well for many years to come.

ABOUT THE AUTHOR

Dr. Patricia Shelton, MD, is a yoga and anatomy teacher trained in medicine. She holds a bachelor's degree in neurobiology and a doctoral degree in medicine. She teaches anatomy in yoga teacher training programs, helping new yoga teachers to understand the body's structure and to learn how to use that knowledge to ensure a safe and effective yoga practice. She also teaches workshops as well as group and private yoga classes. Dr. Patti is passionate about helping others access their own body's intelligence.

You can find out more about Dr. Patti at her website, www.pattisheltonmd.com, where she keeps a blog as well as information about her teaching and retreat schedule.

ACKNOWLEDGMENTS

Many thanks to Laura Mentele, the extraordinarily talented artist who created the illustrations included in this book.

Many thanks also to Eric Mentele, who designed and created the book's beautiful cover.

To the incredible yoga teachers with whom I've had the great fortune to study – especially you, Seong Yoon Lee, Jennifer Hill, Ali Valdez, and Liz Doyle – thank you for giving me the opportunity to receive your wisdom.

Printed in Great Britain
by Amazon